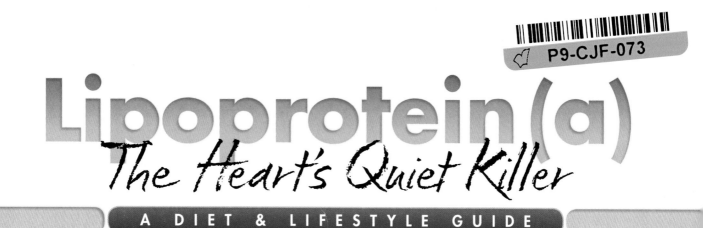

Lipoprotein(a)
The Heart's Quiet Killer

A DIET & LIFESTYLE GUIDE

Joel K. Kahn, MD, FACC

WITH RECIPES BY BEVERLY LYNN BENNETT

BPC

Summertown, Tennessee

Library of Congress Cataloging-in-Publication Data available upon request.

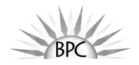

We chose to print this title on responsibly harvested paper stock certified by the Forest Stewardship Council®, an independent auditor of responsible forestry practices. For more information, visit us.fsc.org.

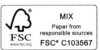

Food photography: Alan Roettinger
Cover photo: Alan Roettinger
Stock photography: 123 RF
Cover and interior design: John Wincek

Printed in Canada

BPC
PO Box 99
Summertown, TN 38483
888-260-8458
bookpubco.com

ISBN: 978-1-57067-387-0

25 24 23 22 21 20   1 2 3 4 5 6 7 8 9

Disclaimer: The information in this book is presented for educational purposes only. It isn't intended to be a substitute for the medical advice of a physician, dietitian, or other health-care professional.

CONTENTS

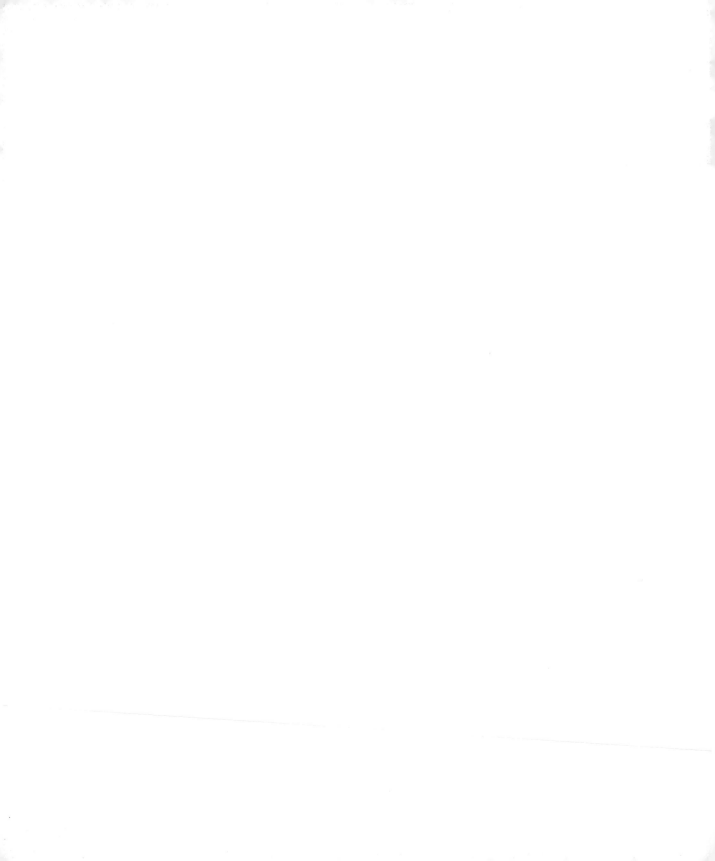

INTRODUCTION

Heart disease is often like a cobra, silent in the bush until it strikes—often lethally. Yet, in the thirty years I've been taking care of patients with suspected or known heart disease, I have seen many advances in our understanding of the prevention, early diagnosis, and possibility for reversing this deadly disease.

Sadly, the current medical community usually does not take an aggressive approach to preventing heart disease. Current medical protocol may help physicians save lives in the middle of crisis situations, such as heart attacks and strokes, but it doesn't provide guidance for preventing these tragedies from happening in the first place. I have fought to keep hospitals, cardiac care units, and operating suites as empty as possible by identifying root causes of heart disease and instituting programs that promote self-care earlier in the course of someone's illness.

In my upstream approach to heart care, I've focused on identifying and counseling individuals found to have an inherited form of cholesterol that's not widely known, yet it is capable of clogging arteries and heart valves: lipoprotein(a), or Lp(a). This cholesterol particle sticks to arteries and valves, and for this reason, Lp(a) is known as "sticky cholesterol." Over one billion people worldwide have elevated levels of Lp(a) and are at risk for early cardiovascular events. While much research about Lp(a) is ongoing and needed, my hope is *Lipoprotein(a): The Heart's Quiet Killer* will serve as a guide for those dealing with this often deadly and unrecognized danger.

What Is Lipoprotein(a)?

Trainers Jillian Michaels and Bob Harper had a big following on the TV show *The Biggest Loser*, where they led severely obese contestants through a program of eating healthy and working out diligently to determine who could lose the most weight. The two trainers appeared glowingly fit, which is why the show's followers were shocked when Bob Harper collapsed in a gym at age fifty-one while on a treadmill. Fortunately, a cardiologist was in the gym at the time and was able to use the automatic external defibrillator the gym kept on hand to shock Harper back to life. Harper was then rushed to a New York hospital and had an emergency procedure to place a stent in one of his heart arteries.

How could one of today's most fit TV personalities suffer a massive heart attack and not have known he was at risk for heart disease? A few months after his heart attack, Harper appeared on the *Dr. Oz Show* and announced that he had a very high Lp(a) level, but he had only learned about it *after* his heart attack. He launched a campaign to raise awareness about heart disease prevention in general and checking Lp(a) levels in particular. He indicated on the show that when he found out about his Lp(a) level, he texted Dr. Oz, who answered back that the presence of LP(a) was great news. Why such great news? Dr. Oz advised him that "now you know what's going on with you and you know what to do."

Bob Harper's story was written up in the *New York Times* as "A Heart Risk Factor Even Doctors Know Little About." Harper said that learning he had elevated Lp(a) made it possible for him to reduce his heart disease risk.

What Is Lipoprotein(a)?

Lp(a) is a complex cholesterol molecule whose presence is determined by genetics. If you inherit Lp(a) from your parents, levels in your blood will reach a plateau at around age two and remain there through to adulthood.

While there are theories about the existence of Lp(a) and why it is elevated in over one billion people, we don't know the exact answers. One interpretation is that having Lp(a) offers an evolutionary advantage to humans (and the few other species that have it) by accelerating wound healing and repairing tissues and blood vessels after a wound or other trauma.

However, Lp(a) can potentially prevent the breakdown of clots and favor their growth. Clotting in critical arteries is the cause of most heart attacks and many strokes, and may lead to narrowing or blockage. This can make it difficult for vital organs to receive the nutrients they need to remain healthy.

Lp(a) varies in size quite a bit due to variations in the apolipoprotein(a) component attached to the LDL cholesterol. There can be a thousand-fold difference in the level of Lp(a) in the blood among various people, which is a much greater variance than there is for LDL cholesterol alone. To confound matters more, Lp(a) doesn't come in one uniform shape but in over forty shapes. This is due to the variation in the size of the apo(a) component of Lp(a), based on the number of something called kringle IV2 loops. Overall, the smaller Lp(a) particles, due to a smaller apo(a) component, are made more rapidly, lead to higher blood levels, and are related more to atherosclerosis and valve damage. The number of kringle loops and the size of the apo(a) component are not routinely measured in most labs outside of research studies.

Lp(a) can cause several types of coronary heart disease, such as heart attack, stroke, peripheral arterial disease, aortic valve disease, and heart failure. Of course, the risk of heart disease from elevated Lp(a) will be even higher if you smoke or have high blood pressure or type 2 diabetes, in addition to other known causes of heart disease. But unlike smoking or diabetes, elevated Lp(a) can influence the risk of blood vessel and heart valve damage from birth, which potentially makes it more deadly than poor lifestyle habits initiated during adulthood.

Many studies have acknowledged the importance of elevated levels of Lp(a) since its identification by Norwegian researchers in 1963. According to a National Heart, Lung, and Blood Institute report published in 2018, an estimated 1.4 billion people globally have elevated Lp(a) levels, representing about 30 percent of the entire population. While an estimated 400 million people worldwide have diabetes, more than three times that number may have accumulated damage to their arteries and valves since infancy from high Lp(a). Elevated Lp(a) levels have been identified in patients with established arterial disease, calcific aortic valve disease, and chronic kidney disease, but it can also occur in people with otherwise normal cholesterol levels.

The Dangers of High Lp(a)

The Canadian-led INTERHEART study of 2004 found that people with high Lp(a) levels (greater than 50 mg/dL) had a risk of heart attacks that was about 1.5 times greater than for people with lower Lp(a) levels. The importance of this study was that this risk was determined to be solely due to Lp(a) and was independent of established heart attack risk factors, including type 2 diabetes, smoking, high blood pressure, and high cholesterol levels.

A study that combined research done from 1970 through 2009 showed that the rates of heart disease in people whose Lp(a) values were in the top third of those measured were 5.6 times higher than those in people with levels in the lowest third. Another analysis published in 2019 indicated that elevated Lp(a) levels were independently associated with an increased risk of overall cardiac events in heart disease patients (although elevated levels didn't seem to increase the risk of death from heart disease). The researchers concluded that measurement of the lipoprotein(a) level has the potential to help people with heart disease—and their health-care providers—determine their level of risk.

Another study done in Denmark in 2009 took a different approach. Instead of measuring the Lp(a) of people who had heart disease, they looked at almost forty thousand people who already had registered Lp(a) levels to see who would develop heart disease (specifically heart attacks) in the future. People with the highest levels of Lp(a) had nearly three times the risk of heart attacks compared to those with the lowest levels. The researchers determined that there was a causal relationship between elevated Lp(a) levels and risk of future heart attacks.

Stroke and Lp(a)

Strokes can be devastating or fatal and should be avoided at all costs. There are many different causes for strokes, but one is a tendency for atherosclerosis and blood clots in blood vessels supplying the brain. Because of this involvement of clotting, there is reason to investigate the role of Lp(a) in the risk of stroke. The carotid arteries are the main sources of blood flow to the brain, and damage to these arteries can create clots that may break off and cause strokes. In 2018, a team of North American researchers examined whether the presence of high Lp(a) levels would correlate with increased risk for stroke. They noted that even though measures were taken to aggressively lower cholesterol levels, higher Lp(a) levels led to more strokes in the individuals they studied.

In 2014, a group of German researchers looked at studies done that year of more than ninety thousand people, comparing those with high Lp(a) levels to those with low Lp(a) levels. The study concluded that the risk for stroke was 1.4 times higher for people with elevated Lp(a) levels. Younger participants with elevated Lp(a) levels had an even higher stroke risk than older participants. In 2016, US researchers came to a similar conclusion about stroke risk in young to middle-aged people with elevated Lp(a).

Other Heart Disease Risks

Severe thickening of the aortic valve leading into the heart (known as calcific aortic valve disease) is less prevalent than heart attack or stroke, but it still affects a large number of people—killing approximately 150,000 a year. The risk of dying from a blocked valve is 25 percent at one year after a diagnosis and 50 percent at two years unless action is taken to correct it. Lp(a) will cause progressive calcification and malfunction of the aortic valve in ways that cholesterol will not. Lp(a) levels in people with this disease are not routinely measured, but studies indicate how important this information would be for both patients and doctors. A recent study in Denmark following almost seventy-eight thousand people found that elevated Lp(a) levels were associated with an increasing risk of calcific aortic valve disease that was as much as three times higher than the general population. Gene studies at McGill University in Montreal also show a relationship between Lp(a) levels and calcific aortic valve disease.

Traditional risk assessment for heart disease in women may not be as accurate as it is in men. Chicago researchers discovered that high Lp(a) levels were a better predictor of risk for cardiovascular disease in many women, even when those women were assessed as having low to normal risk from other factors. This makes a strong case for ensuring that otherwise healthy women have their Lp(a) levels measured. A Swedish study of almost three hundred women under sixty-five years old found that the risk for heart disease increased two to three times in women with elevated LP(a), regardless of whether the women had gone through menopause or not. This is an important finding for premenopausal women, who may think their active hormone levels protect them against heart disease.

It's also important to note the possible risk that Lp(a) can pose for children, since levels can be as high at age two as they are later in life. Although studies have not measured Lp(a) levels against actual health events, this is more because lipoprotein is not routinely measured in children or adults and doesn't reflect how important a problem it can be—especially if either parent has had an unexpected heart disease incident. Because the danger of stroke is a potential risk for young people, it's particularly important that they avoid lifestyle habits that increase the risk for heart disease overall, such as smoking, overeating, and being sedentary.

Residual Risk: Why Lp(a) Matters So Much

Some patients who have heart disease or are at risk for future heart disease can do all the right things—take the correct medications and adopt healthful lifestyle measures—and still end up having a heart attack, stroke, heart stent procedure, or bypass. They may not even survive that event. How can this happen? The ongoing danger of experiencing health problems when conventional therapies are used is termed "residual risk." The concept mainly comes from research trials with statin medications. Although prescribing a statin may be appropriate for some patients and may lower cholesterol levels and heart attack rates by 20–40 percent, the majority of the risk for heart disease still remains. This does not imply that prescribing a statin is not of some benefit or that they should be stopped.

Even when LDL cholesterol is controlled in a normal range, Lp(a) may be a marker for identifying and evaluating the residual cardiovascular risk. Recent research has evaluated the role of Lp(a) in residual risk for heart disease patients. A team of investigators developed a system to estimate this risk in over three thousand adults with heart disease who were on statin therapy. They determined that the strongest predictor of recurrent heart events, despite statin therapy, was elevated Lp(a). Therefore, knowing your Lp(a) level is a crucial component of knowing your overall health status.

Why Aren't Lp(a) Levels Routinely Tested?

Unfortunately, the increased risk caused by elevated Lp(a) has not yet gained recognition from most practicing physicians and health-care providers. Why have most people not heard about Lp(a) and have not had it measured on their visits to their health-care team? The answer reminds me of that song in *Fiddler on the Roof:* "Tradition." The way we assess heart disease today is not much different from how it was assessed forty to fifty years ago.

For example, the American Heart Association has developed and promoted a list called "Life's Simple 7," which lists risk factors that individuals can avoid to reduce their chances of developing heart attacks, strokes, and other important forms of heart disease. These actions include not smoking, obtaining regular fitness checks, making the best dietary choices, maintaining an optimal weight, and measuring and managing blood pressure, blood sugar, and blood cholesterol. Attaining just five of these seven goals has been shown to reduce the risk of heart-related deaths by 78 percent compared with achieving none of the seven goals.

However, when assessments are made of how many people achieve all seven of these preventive health methods, the number is shockingly low, primarily due to how few people eat a healthy diet. While Life's Simple 7 is useful and something I teach in my preventive clinic, there are really more than seven factors to focus on, and elevated Lp(a) is the most common risk not measured routinely. There is even a foundation that hosts a website to educate the public about Lp(a), but most people are unaware of it. (See the resources on page 137.)

Also, Lp(a) is only found in a few species: humans, old-world nonhuman primates (such as the rhesus monkey and baboon), and the European hedgehog. Why humans are a part of such a small and unusual group of carriers of Lp(a) is not yet known. However, Lp(a) is not found in animals commonly used to research human diseases, such as rats, mice, and rabbits, so studies that use these animals to learn more about heart disease in humans will not uncover Lp(a) as a contributing factor.

What Are Normal and High-Risk Levels of Lp(a)?

The standards for measuring Lp(a) levels are not always consistent; sometimes they are measured in milligrams per deciliter (mg/dl) and in other instances in nanomoles per liter (nmol/L). Although these systems are measuring different qualities, a high measurement of one type usually correlates to a high measurement of another type. Race and ethnicity can also influence the level of Lp(a) found in certain people. In one analysis, for example, average Lp(a) levels in Caucasian Americans were less than one-third of those in African Americans.

In general, Lp(a) levels greater than 30 mg/dl are reported as abnormal, but some practitioners feel that only levels greater than 50 mg/dl are what should be considered abnormal. When reported by particle size, a level greater than 75 nmol/L is reported as abnormal, while a level greater than 100–125 nmol/L is considered high risk. Currently, the same upper limit is used for African Americans, but the data does indicate a higher average level in large populations overall. I have many patients in my clinic with Lp(a) levels in the 300s, 400s, and even 500s, measured either by mass or number of particles.

Who Should Have Their Lp(a) Tested?

Few people receive routine Lp(a) testing, at least in the United States. This is likely to change with the increasing research on the importance of Lp(a) for determining residual risk for heart disease. The National Lipid Association produced a scientific statement that recommends who should be tested:

- First-degree relatives (parents, children, siblings) who have experienced early heart disease events (under sixty-five years of age for female relatives and fifty-five years for male relatives)
- People with a personal history of premature atherosclerosis or cardiovascular disease
- Those with high cholesterol levels, such as an LDL level greater than 190 mg/dl

Other reasons for testing include the following:

- To aid in the discussion about risk and whether a statin is needed (primarily for people age forty to seventy-five with lower risk)
- To evaluate why a statin did not lower LDL as much as expected
- To screen family members in cases of severely elevated cholesterol
- To identify people at risk for progression of coronary artery disease

The most recent guidelines regarding testing for Lp(a) come from the European Atherosclerosis Society. The society went beyond the National Lipid Association in stating that the measurement of Lp(a) should be considered at least once in each adult's lifetime to identify those with very high inherited Lp(a) levels (greater than 180 mg/dl or 430 nmol/L). These people may have a lifetime risk of cardiovascular disease equivalent to the risk of having a genetic defect associated with dangerously high cholesterol levels (heterozygous familial hyperlipidemia, or HeFH). I favor this additional indication for measurement of Lp(a), and I do test everyone at my clinic for Lp(a) at least once.

Lab Tests for Risk Assessment in Addition to Lp(a)

Although not universally embraced, one path to further lower the risk of cardiovascular disease is a more extensive lab evaluation searching for both traditional risk factors (such as glucose and cholesterol levels) and additional risk factors. In my clinic, I use extensive lab analyses. The list of laboratory tests that you might request from your health-care provider or order directly from laboratory providers is potentially quite long, and these tests could be expensive. The following list of laboratory tests was compiled by the Cleveland Clinic, and I agree with it:

BASIC LABORATORY TESTS TO EVALUATE CARDIOVASCULAR RISK

- Lipids: total cholesterol (TC)
- Triglycerides (TG)
- High-density lipoprotein (HDL) cholesterol
- LDL cholesterol, calculated and direct
- Complete blood count with differential (CBC)
- Hemoglobin A1c (HgA1c), to assess blood sugar levels over the last two to three months
- Fasting glucose (also called fasting blood sugar)
- Fasting insulin

ADVANCED LABORATORY BLOOD TESTS FOR CARDIOVASCULAR DISEASE

- Lipoprotein(a)
- Fibrinogen
- Apolipoprotein B or ApoB (another way to assess LDL cholesterol)
- NMR LipoProfile (provides cholesterol particle numbers and size)
- Alanine aminotransferase (ALT) and aspartate transaminase (AST), for liver health
- High-sensitivity C-reactive protein (hs-CRP), for inflammation
- Thyroid-stimulating hormone (TSH), free T4, and free T3, to assess thyroid health
- Brain natriuretic peptide (BNP or NT-proBNP), a protein in the heart that's released when there is strain on the heart

- Myeloperoxidase (MPO) and Lp-PLA2, to also assess inflammation
- Vitamin D levels

There are other lab tests available, including genetic markers, such as ApoE and MTHFR, GGT for liver toxicity, and heavy metal toxin levels. You can discuss these with your health team.

Detecting Cardiovascular and Aortic Valve Disease When There Are No Symptoms

If there is one thing that I am most proud of in my thirty-plus years of practicing cardiology, it is the thousands if not millions of people I have educated about the importance of identifying cardiovascular disease at an early stage, when it has been previously undetected. Calcific aortic valve disease (CAVD) is often found during a physical examination when a murmur (an unusual sound during blood flow) is heard using a stethoscope over the heart and upper chest. By the time a murmur is detected, the aortic valve has been inflamed, has thickened, and has filled with calcium deposits for months to years. CAVD usually has few to no symptoms until it is far advanced. A more definitive way to detect and evaluate CAVD is echocardiography, or ultrasound of the heart. About 1 percent of people are born with a defect in the aortic valve and can develop CAVD at a much earlier age. Finally, more advanced cardiac imaging, such as MRIs, CTs, and cardiac catheterization, can identify and quantify the amount of CAVD you may have, but these are not screening examinations. I suggest that you ask your health provider during your next visit whether you have a heart murmur.

Heart disease in general is a much bigger challenge to detect, as it is far more frequent than CAVD. It can go undetected for years until it manifests suddenly with a heart attack, stroke, or even death. Sadly, most of the medical community currently does not screen for silent heart disease, even though there are ways to do this that are simple and inexpensive.

In 2005, I learned of the Society for Heart Attack Prevention and Eradication (SHAPE Society) and adopted its approach for heart disease testing and treatment. The SHAPE Society has been a vocal proponent for addressing cardiovascular risk in asymptomatic individuals through the imaging of arteries. The two ways the society recommends evaluating for silent damage to arteries are a coronary artery calcium CT scan (CACS) or a carotid intima-medial

Heart Disease—A Primer

Cardiovascular disease is the number one cause of death globally and in the US. More people die annually from this condition than from any other cause, and more than 80 percent of these deaths are from heart attacks and strokes. Cardiovascular disease is also the leading cause of death for most racial or ethnic groups in the United States, including African Americans, Hispanics, and whites. For Asian Americans, Pacific Islanders, American Indians, and Alaska Natives, heart disease is second only to cancer. Consider these statistics:

- Cardiovascular disease is the leading cause of death for men in the United States, killing approximately 321,000 men in 2013. That's one in every four male deaths.

- Half of the men who die suddenly of cardiovascular disease had no previous symptoms.

- Between 70 and 90 percent of sudden cardiac death events occur in men.

- Despite increases in awareness over the past decades, only about 50 percent of women recognize that atherosclerosis (hardening and narrowing of the arteries) is their number one risk for death.

- Cardiovascular disease is the leading cause of death for women of all ethnic groups in the United States, killing almost 300,000 women in 2017—or about one in every five female deaths.

Cardiovascular disease is not the only deadly consequence related to high lipoprotein levels; stroke is as well. You may not always be able to tell whether you've had a stroke. Some strokes are symptomatic, affecting speech or the loss of function of one side of the body; others may be identified only on imaging, such as a brain CT or MRI scan. When considered separately from other cardiovascular diseases, stroke ranks fifth among all causes of death in the US, killing approximately 142,000 people a year. According to data from 2005, stroke was also a leading cause of serious long-term disability in the US.

Even though there are challenges to lowering high lipoprotein levels, you can still reduce your risk for health problems caused by Lp(a) by following the guidelines for reducing heart disease in general. Several medical conditions and lifestyle choices put people at a higher risk for heart disease, including the following:

- High blood pressure
- Diabetes
- Having a parent or sibling who developed heart disease at an early age
- Overweight and obesity
- Tobacco use
- A diet of processed foods and meats that is also low in fruits and vegetables
- Physical inactivity
- Excessive alcohol use

Most cardiovascular diseases can be prevented by addressing the behavioral risk factors listed above. There are also conditions that may cause inflammation and other conditions that can lead to cardiovascular diseases, including these:

- Abdominal obesity
- Breast cancer treatment
- Erectile dysfunction
- Gestational diabetes
- Gout
- Gum disease
- Hirsutism (facial hair growth in women)
- Lupus
- Migraine headaches
- Oligomenorrhea (changes in menstrual cycles)
- Osteoporosis
- Secondary exposure to nicotine use (such as secondhand smoke)
- Polycystic ovaries
- Preeclampsia
- Psoriasis
- Psychosocial issues, such as depression, anxiety, or stress
- Rheumatoid arthritis
- Sleep problems

thickness (CIMT) ultrasound. The CT scan takes under a minute, often costs less than one hundred dollars, involves no injection of medications, and is widely available. The dose of radiation is on par with a mammogram. The CIMT is less widely available but does not require X-rays and is an exam I do in my clinic.

After the tests are done, the true level or risk can be determined and treatment, according to the individual risk level, can be offered. The good news is that not all adults with elevated Lp(a) have cardiovascular disease, and these tests may be perfectly normal. Both the CACS and the CIMT allow a measure of the true "arterial age" of a patient early in his or her course of aortic disease. There is an online calculator available (see the resources on page 137) that incorporates the results of the CACS, historical features, and lab values into a ten-year assessment of the risk for a heart attack or stroke. I use this number with my patients both to educate them on their risk and to plan therapy, and it has been extremely helpful.

Traditional and Alternative Treatments for Lipoprotein(a)

Studies have been done on a number of medications and supplements to determine their ability to lower cholesterol in general and Lp(a) levels specifically. The results for many of these substances have been mixed, but there are a few that show promise.

Statins and Lp(a)

Statins are a class of prescription medications that were introduced for use in the US in 1987. Statin medications block the activity of an enzyme in the liver that helps form cholesterol, and they can reduce blood cholesterol levels by up to 50 percent. It is standard practice for doctors to prescribe a statin medication to anyone who has been diagnosed with cardiovascular disease in order to prevent future adverse events, so it would be ideal if statins also lowered Lp(a). The overall consensus is that they do not.

Several studies show that statins may actually raise Lp(a) levels. For example, a recent review of the studies done on Lp(a) stated that statins tended to increase Lp(a) levels, possibly contributing to the risk of heart problems observed in people with those high levels. If statins do increase Lp(a), that is concerning. In a formal research study of 591 patients treated for twenty-four weeks with statins in combination with other lipid-lowering medications, measurements revealed an increase in levels of Lp(a). As part of the research, a review of the medical literature indicated that statins increased Lp(a) by about 11 percent. Some studies show an increase of more than twice that. However, we simply don't have enough information to know the impact of statins on Lp(a) levels over the long term and rarely would taking a statin elevate normal Lp(a) metrics into a high-risk range. Major studies of statins demonstrated reduced risks for CVD events even in those with elevated Lp(a) levels.

The only exceptions might be in individuals with the genetic cholesterol disorder called heterozygous familial hyperlipidemia, or HeFH. People with this disorder produce very high levels of LDL cholesterol from birth, and often very high levels of Lp(a) as well. HeFH may be inherited by as many as 1 in 250 people, making it far less common than Lp(a); however, this group may respond to statin therapy in a more significant manner than the general public. A Dutch study showed an approximate 20 percent decrease in Lp(a) levels in people with this disorder when they were given either atorvastatin or simvastatin.

In general, however, statins seem to have a role to play when someone has high Lp(a) levels, if for nothing else than to reduce heart disease risk from elevated LDL cholesterol. While it hasn't been definitively established that statins should be prescribed routinely for people with elevated Lp(a), the goal of achieving ideal cardiovascular health (which includes lowering LDL cholesterol levels through diet, lifestyle, and possibly medications and supplements) is strongly supported. The use of statins must be considered case by case.

Other Medications

The case for taking a low-dose aspirin to reduce Lp(a) levels is not clear, but there have been cases in which it was shown to have a significant positive effect. Therefore, it seems wise to take an adult low-strength aspirin (around 75 mg) if your Lp(a) is moderately to severely elevated, particularly if you had a coronary artery calcium score (CACS) over 100, which is considered abnormal. (See page 137 for more information on coronary artery calcium scores.)

Fibrates are prescription medications that have been used for decades to decrease levels of cholesterol and triglycerides. Researchers from Australia examined studies that assessed the effects of fibrate medications, along with statin drugs, on Lp(a) levels. The ability to lower Lp(a) with fibrates was greater overall than with statins, but improvement was small. In studies, fibrate therapy alone had a greater influence on lowering Lp(a) than it did when it was combined with a statin. Neither fibrates nor statins promise much benefit for lowering Lp(a) levels effectively.

Ezetimibe is a prescription medication that lowers cholesterol levels by inhibiting the absorption of intestinal cholesterol by a specific receptor in the small intestine. Ezetimibe may be used alone or in combination with a statin or other agents. Data from ten randomized trials, including over five thousand subjects treated with either ezetimibe or a placebo, showed that the medication had no effect on Lp(a) levels. That held true whether ezetimibe was used by itself or combined with other agents. But its effectiveness at lowering LDL cholesterol might make it worth considering for individuals with high Lp(a) and high cholesterol.

Niacin (vitamin B$_3$) has long been viewed as effective in reducing cholesterol levels, and it has also been considered for Lp(a) reduction therapy. As with many other substances, the results for lowering Lp(a) with niacin have been mixed. In my clinic, I often opt to use niacin combined with lifestyle measures for my patients with high Lp(a), even though there is no definitive long-term outcome data to demonstrate reduced events and niacin failed to meet its primary endpoint in three major clinical trials. There can be side effects from niacin use—including flushing, rash, a rise in blood sugar, and muscle aches—and these are taken into account in my discussions with patients as we weigh possible benefits versus risks.

In fairness, using niacin on its own has only been studied in individuals with high cholesterol and not specifically in people with elevated Lp(a), so it is simply not known if niacin alone reduces plaque and the incidence of cardiovascular disease. There are reports of combining extended-release niacin with omega-3 fatty acid supplements to lower Lp(a) levels. In a small study of people with high Lp(a) who followed this regimen, the overall reduction in Lp(a) was 23 percent in individuals who completed the study.

Nutraceuticals and Lp(a)

There are a number of reports on nutritional supplements and vitamins and their impact on Lp(a) levels. The fancy word for these agents is nutraceuticals (as opposed to pharmaceuticals). A recent review identified coffee, CoQ10, and L-carnitine as hopeful for lowering Lp(a).

Coffee

Coffee is known to reduce plasma lipids (such as triglycerides) and cholesterol. However, a handful of studies on the effect of coffee drinking showed either a small decrease in Lp(a) or no effect. One study showed that Lp(a) was somewhat elevated in chronic consumers of boiled coffee, but less so for drinkers of filtered coffee.

CoQ10

Coenzyme Q10, also known as CoQ10, is a nutrient that is manufactured naturally in the body, but levels start to decrease once people are over age forty. CoQ10 functions as a powerful antioxidant to prevent damage to cells and organs. Evidence exists that CoQ10 supports healthy blood pressure, relieves migraines, and helps to maintain healthy heart function even in the advanced stages of congestive heart failure.

Supplemental CoQ10 has been studied to see if it will lower Lp(a). In 1999, a study using a specific type of CoQ10 gel produced a 31 percent drop in Lp(a) levels. Along with those changes, the use of CoQ10 also resulted in an increase in HDL levels and a reduction in blood sugar. (Further study is needed to determine if other types of CoQ10 preparations would produce the same response.) An interesting study was performed on patients receiving dialysis for end-stage kidney disease, which can elevate the risk for cardiovascular events. The patients were given either CoQ10 or L-carnitine (more information on this follows), or both, or neither. All three groups that received some form of supplementation demonstrated significant drops in Lp(a) levels, about 20 percent.

A recent review article consolidated the findings on CoQ10 and Lp(a) levels. CoQ10 supplementation showed a slight reduction of Lp(a), but the rate of reduction rose in people with higher levels (greater than 30 mg/dL) of Lp(a) at the start of the studies. Interestingly, CoQ10 is not effective in reducing cholesterol levels.

L-carnitine

L-carnitine is a nutrient derived from the amino acid lysine. It is available widely as a supplement, usually in capsule form. There has been a tremendous amount of research on the role of L-carnitine in health and disease. In 2000, reports appeared about the potential for supplemental L-carnitine to lower elevated Lp(a) levels. One study of thirty-six people with elevated Lp(a) showed a 12 percent reduction in Lp(a) after receiving L-carnitine supplementation. A more recent study reviewing previous work on Lp(a) levels showed significant reduction following supplementation with L-carnitine.

However, a new concern has surfaced about the role of L-carnitine in raising levels of a substance called trimethylamine N-oxide (TMAO), which has been shown to promote atherosclerosis and scarring of the heart muscle. TMAO appears in the bloodstream after a person eats red meat, and the

L-carnitine found in red meat has been identified as a precursor to producing TMAO. A recent study done in collaboration with the Cleveland Clinic showed how L-carnitine supplements lead to a marked rise in TMAO levels. I've seen similar results in lab tests I've prescribed for my patients, so I monitor their use of L-carnitine supplements and reduce or eliminate them from their treatment plans if the patients' TMAO levels become high.

Vitamin C

Linus Pauling, PhD, is famous for his biochemical research focused on the role of vitamin C in health and disease. He identified that only a few species (of which humans are one) are incapable of synthesizing vitamin C from glucose. We are completely dependent on diet to provide vitamin C. One of vitamin C's many functions is to help produce collagen, which holds arteries, skin, and organs together. If we don't eat enough foods with vitamin C, we can experience scurvy, a disease that weakens collagen and can result in bleeding gums, skin problems, and ruptured blood vessels. Humans may require much higher amounts of vitamin C for optimal health and the prevention of heart disease than are currently recommended.

Properties of Lp(a) that are shared with vitamin C are the acceleration of wound healing and other cell-repair mechanisms, the strengthening of the extracellular matrix (such as in blood vessels), and the prevention of cholesterol damage, or peroxidation. Pauling noted that humans are at a rare biological intersection, as some of us can synthesize Lp(a) but not vitamin C, so he hypothesized that Lp(a) might be present in humans as a replacement for vitamin C. Studies in 2015, done by a former student of Pauling's, suggest that the tendency of Lp(a) to stick to valves and vessel walls may be prevented by increasing the intake of vitamin C and lysine. Whether you increase your vitamin C intake through diet or supplements, the health of your arteries will improve due to enhanced collagen formation.

Other Supplements

Garlic and ginkgo biloba are two nutraceuticals that have been used to protect against heart disease, and although studies show favorable results when they're used for heart disease in general, these substances haven't been shown to lower Lp(a) levels specifically. Although there's information that suggests that a combination of vitamin C and lysine might prevent atherosclerosis, there is no definitive data to show that it reduces Lp(a) in humans. Omega-3 fatty acids have also been shown to be beneficial in treating or preventing heart disease, but their effect on Lp(a) levels is inconclusive.

Hormone Replacement Therapy and Lp(a)

One of the many reasons women undertake hormone replacement therapy (HRT) after the onset of menopause is because it's been shown to reduce heart disease risk. HRT has also been shown to reduce Lp(a) levels, but it's not clear if this reduction also leads to reduced risk. There's very little information on the effect of testosterone replacement therapy in men on Lp(a) levels, aside from some older studies. Because of complications that can result from hormone replacement therapy, the risks versus benefits should be weighed before doctors recommend it either for anti-aging or to lower Lp(a) levels.

Advanced Therapies for Lp(a)

After years of investigation and large clinical trials, a new class of prescription agents that lower LDL cholesterol, called PCSK9 inhibitors, was approved in 2015. These agents require an injection under the skin twice a month. PCSK9 inhibitors cause more LDL to be removed from the bloodstream and can lower Lp(a) levels by about 25 percent by reducing the synthesis of apo(a). The downside of treatments with PCSK9 inhibitors is that they are expensive ($5,000 to $6,000, depending on insurance coverage) and produce uncertain results. Some studies show that they may be more effective for people with high levels of Lp(a).

One of the most aggressive therapies for elevated Lp(a) levels is also one of the most effective. Apheresis, or "taking away," is a process in which a patient's blood is filtered through a machine similar to what is used for hemodialysis. The treatment separates out a component of the blood and returns the rest to the patient. One form of treatment is known as LDL apheresis; it uses a cartridge filter to bind to LDL cholesterol, causing dramatic and rapid drops in levels of LDL in the blood. Patients have an IV port (such as those put in place for cancer chemotherapy or dialysis) inserted or have an IV inserted during each treatment. They then spend several hours twice a month having their blood filtered through the apparatus.

Apheresis has been used for patients with a family history of high cholesterol and for patients with either symptoms of heart disease and an LDL cholesterol level over 200 mg or LDL cholesterol levels over 300 mg without known disease. Children and teenagers have also been treated this way. Side effects, including low blood pressure and issues related to the IV catheter, are common over repeated treatments.

The largest studies on apheresis have been done in Germany and have shown a 70 percent reduction in cardiac events, and up to a 90 percent reduction in some cases. A study in London also reported a rapid improvement in heart disease symptoms (such as angina) with apheresis, as well as improved stamina and overall quality of life. The same group reported improvements in clotting and blood flow after apheresis, along with a reduction in inflammatory markers.

Developing and sustaining an apheresis clinic is very costly and labor intensive. I have referred a few patients to these clinics over the course of my thirty-year career. The introduction of PCSK9 inhibitors—particularly when combined as needed with statins and ezetimibe, along with diet and lifestyle—has reduced the demand for apheresis. The FH Foundation website (see page 137) lists centers that perform apheresis.

Research on new medications to lower lipoprotein levels continues. One promising therapy called antisense oligonucleotide (ASO) introduces a substance into the body that will turn off the gene that creates elevated Lp(a). Researchers are testing different doses and dose frequencies to find the most effective levels in persons with the highest of Lp(a) levels at high risk for events. A recent study showed decreased Lp(a) levels up to 80 percent in some individuals, especially those who had weekly treatments. Further trials are planned, and the journey to approve antisense oligonucleotides for use will still require at least a few more years to complete trials and be presented to the FDA. Whether the therapy stabilizes or reduces plaques in carotid and coronary arteries and whether it lowers the rates of heart attacks, strokes, and death is hoped for but not yet proven. If it is ultimately approved, it likely will be limited at first to the highest-risk patients with advanced CVD.

3 Total Heart Lp(a) Plan

here is definitive proof that heart disease is reversible. This is crucial for patients with elevated Lp(a), because the same pattern of diet and lifestyle that should be adopted to minimize the effects of heart disease overall will also minimize the effects of elevated Lp(a).

The Effects of Lifestyle on Lp(a) Levels

In 1997, a study was published that investigated the diets of fifty-eight men and women with elevated Lp(a) levels. The diets contained different types and amounts of fats, such as trans fats, saturated fats, and oleic acid (the predominant fat in olive oil). The diet with saturated fat lowered Lp(a) levels by 8–11 percent. Compared to the oleic diet, the diet with trans fat had no adverse overall effect on Lp(a) levels. However, those study participants with high levels (30 mg/dL or higher) of Lp(a) had a slight increase (5 percent) in Lp(a) levels relative to those on the diets with oleic acid and moderate trans fat. The researchers concluded that the amount of saturated fatty acids commonly found in the typical US diet in the 1990s consistently decreased Lp(a) concentrations by a small amount. (Trans fats have largely been removed from US food production since this study was completed.) There also was no group of study participants who were treated with diets low in saturated fats and cholesterol, such as a whole-foods plant-based diet. The long-term consequences (including accelerated atherosclerosis) of a diet high in saturated fats would make this way of eating inadvisable.

By 2014, more data became available regarding diet and Lp(a). In a feeding study, 155 individuals were given DASH-type healthy diets—rich in either carbohydrates, protein, or unsaturated fat—for six weeks each. Plasma Lp(a) concentrations were assessed at the start of the study and again after each diet had been completed. All of the diets increased Lp(a) levels by a small amount,

2–5 mg/dl. Although the study was not done exclusively with people who had elevated Lp(a), the data was disappointing with regard to the role of diet and the management of Lp(a).

The most exciting data evaluating the role of diet in the therapy of elevated Lp(a) comes from a four-week appraisal of plant-based diets on blood levels. Overweight and obese individuals with elevated LDL cholesterol consumed a plant-based diet for four weeks. Significant reductions were observed for levels of Lp(a)—as much as 32 nmol/L—along with other measures of cholesterol, such as LDL cholesterol. Measures of inflammation also improved on the plant-based diet. The authors concluded that this type of diet can substantially reduce Lp(a). In light of the data collected over a span of more than fifty years showing that a whole-foods plant-based diet can reverse established heart disease, I advise all my patients with elevated Lp(a) to adopt such a diet.

An interesting study evaluated the role of adding flaxseeds to the diet and measured Lp(a) levels before and after this addition. Sixty-two individuals got either 40 grams a day of baked products containing ground flaxseeds or matching products containing wheat bran for ten weeks. During this time, both LDL cholesterol and Lp(a) levels fell for participants consuming the flaxseeds, with the reduction in Lp(a) averaging 14 percent.

There is agreement among the experts that controlling the risk factors for heart disease in general (other than Lp(a) levels) is one way to reduce the risk of cardiovascular disease. There are other nutrition strategies that extend beyond the proven benefits of a whole-foods plant-based diet. One approach to lowering LDL cholesterol that was the rage in the 1980s involved oat bran. Oat bran is the outer lining of the oat kernel that's left after the inedible outer shell is removed. Studies have demonstrated that oat bran is capable of lowering LDL cholesterol levels when used on a consistent basis. For example, one study examined two diets for two weeks administered in succession to twelve volunteers. The first diet included a breakfast of cornflakes; the following diet contained an oat-bran cereal that provided 25 grams of oat bran. Total cholesterol was 5 percent lower and LDL cholesterol levels were 8 percent lower on the oat-bran diet than on the cornflake diet..

In a double-blind, randomized study, twenty-four young adults either followed a low-fiber diet or took a diet supplement with 100 grams of oat bran daily. During the study, the participants switched diets. Total cholesterol decreased by 14 percent when they were on the oat-bran diet compared with 4 percent while eating the low-fiber diet. Several factors that elevate the formation of blood clots also decreased during the oat-bran diet. I advise all of my patients to include oat bran in their diets to lower LDL cholesterol, whether or not they have elevated Lp(a).

Focusing on Total Heart Health

Researchers in England evaluated the role of ideal cardiovascular health on the long-term outcome of people with elevated Lp(a). They used the American Heart Association's "Life's Simple 7" scoring system, which evaluates body mass index (the ratio of height versus weight), diet, physical activity, smoking status, blood pressure, and blood glucose and cholesterol levels. Together, positive measures of these indicators classify someone as having ideal cardiovascular health. Body mass index was considered ideal if it was lower than 25, intermediate if it was between 25 and 30, or poor if it was greater than 30. A healthy diet score was based on intake of five dietary components: fruits and vegetables, fish, whole grains, low sodium intake, and low consumption of sugar-sweetened beverages.

More than fourteen thousand people participated in this study (known as the EPIC-Norfolk study.) Their heart health was ranked as ideal, intermediate, or poor based on the scoring used to evaluate the seven health indicators. Almost two thousand of the participants had a cardiovascular event in the twelve years following the initial measurements. Among participants with high serum Lp(a) levels (greater than 50 mg/dl), those with the highest cardiovascular health score had only one-third the risk of developing cardiovascular disease compared to participants who had the lowest indicator scores. That's a nearly 70 percent reduction in adverse heart health events. The message is clear. As the authors wrote, "Ideal cardiovascular health could substantially reduce CVD risk associated with high Lp(a) levels."

It is important to stress the benefits of a regular exercise program for heart and vascular health and to reduce the risk of adverse events in patients with elevated Lp(a). There is little information, however, regarding the specific effects of exercise on lowering elevated Lp(a). A review article evaluated the available data and found that just moderate physical activity and an improvement in diet alone do not appear to significantly lower Lp(a). But this should not discourage people with high Lp(a) from doing whatever they can to improve their overall heart health. If anything, there is a clear imperative that individuals with high Lp(a) should do all they can to adopt healthy lifestyle measures.

The Case for Plant-Based Diets

No matter what current and upcoming therapies you select for elevated Lp(a), the best approach for avoiding cardiovascular disease will always be a healthy lifestyle. While adequate sleep, a regular fitness routine, stress management, avoidance of smoking, being connected to your community, and having a purpose in life are all critically important, a diet plan for life remains the most important daily decision to lower the risk of cardiovascular disease. Over seventy years of data leads to a single conclusion about which diet provides the greatest protection: eating whole plant foods favors a youthful cardiovascular system, and eating processed foods and animal-derived foods (meat, fish, dairy, eggs) favors an increased risk of suffering the consequences of stroke, heart attack, and aortic valve disease. This is true whether or not you have elevated Lp(a), but it is even more important if you inherited this sticky cholesterol. That is why all the recipes in this book are entirely plant-based and do not include animal products.

It's well known that, in general, animal products are not as health promoting as plant-based foods. One of the reasons is the total absence of fiber in animal-based foods. Cholesterol is only found in animal products, and the odds of eating a higher amount of saturated fats are greater when eating these foods as well. (Coconut and palm oils are among the few saturated fats found in plant-based foods, but they are highly processed, so it's best to avoid them.) Phytonutrients are protective substances found only in plants. You may have heard of two particular phytonutrients—sulforaphane (available in raw cruciferous vegetables, such as broccoli and broccoli sprouts) and resveratrol (found in wine and peanuts)—but there are hundreds of others.

Early Research on Plant-Based Diets

Research into the protective qualities of plant-based foods began in the Los Angeles clinic of internal medicine physician Lester Morrison. He was caring for heart disease patients and survivors of heart attacks in the 1940s, a time when therapies for these conditions were nearly nonexistent. Morrison designed a dietary plan for his heart patients that omitted rich foods, such as cream, butter, and other full-fat dairy products; glandular organs; and egg yolks; as well as olives, nuts, avocados, and oils. He tracked the patients who followed this diet and compared them to patients who did not alter their diets. His results were published in a well-respected medical journal in 1951 and showed that deaths were reduced more than 50 percent after eight years, and in the low-fat diet group, were reduced even more after twelve years.

Another pioneer in cardiovascular therapy was former aerospace engineer Nathan Pritikin, who failed an exercise stress test he took after learning that his cholesterol was over 300 mg/dl. After reading several articles on optimal lifestyles for health, Pritikin designed a plant-based regimen rich in beans and low in fat and combined it with walking. He was able to lower his cholesterol by nearly 200 points (at a time when there were no drug therapies for high cholesterol), and slowly his stress test results returned to normal. He began counseling people with heart disease, obesity, hypertension, and adult diabetes, and he observed stunning examples of reversal. That inspired him to write *The Pritikin Diet*, which became an international best seller and earned him an appearance on *60 Minutes*. He opened the Pritikin Center in Santa Monica, California, and it continues to this day in Miami, Florida, where it is known as the Pritikin Longevity Center + Spa.

After three weeks in practice as an interventional cardiologist, my career changed on July 21, 1990. On that day, *The Lancet,* a widely respected medical journal, published a study that concluded that diet and lifestyle could reverse the presence of heart plaques. Dean Ornish, MD, and his co-researchers debunked the standard belief that heart disease was irreversible. They studied the effects of a low-fat, plant-based diet along with stress reduction, fitness, and social support for patients diagnosed with heart blockages. The team demonstrated that patients who adhered to this lifestyle program not only felt better, but that their subsequent coronary angiograms showed reduced narrowing of their arteries as well. Ornish and his colleagues followed these research patients for longer periods of time, and further testing showed even more health improvements, helping to avoid expensive hospitalizations and treatments.

A similar program at the Cleveland Clinic Foundation was led by heart surgeon Caldwell Esselstyn. He monitored patients with advanced heart disease who converted to totally plant-based diets without added oils, nuts, or other high-fat plant-based foods. Esselstyn documented shrinking and reversal of heart blockages in these patients. The data he accumulated on improved symptoms, sexual function, stress test results, hospital visits, and fewer coronary lesions proved that heart disease could be reversed.

Recent Research on Plant-Based Diets

Since the work of these early researchers, there have been a number of large studies that have compared the health of people eating diets high in plant-based foods to people eating diets high in meat and animal-based foods. The PREDIMED study conducted in Spain was a novel experiment in which more than seven thousand people at high risk for cardiovascular disease were assigned to three diets, and their progress was followed for nearly five years. They filled out extensive food questionnaires to keep track of which foods they consumed over that time. Fruits, vegetables, nuts, cereals, legumes, olive oil, and potatoes were considered healthy choices, while butter, eggs, fish, dairy, and meats were negatively scored. The individuals who ate the greatest amount of plant-based foods had a 40 percent reduction in their risk of dying from heart disease.

A recent study published in the *Journal of the American Heart Association* followed over twelve thousand people from 1987 to 2016, and their diets were assessed according to the amount of plant- and animal-based foods they ate. Nutritious plant-based diets provided a lower risk of cardiovascular disease and overall death rates by 18 to 32 percent compared to diets high in animal-based foods.

The Adventist Health Study was established in 1958 after data indicated that Seventh-day Adventist residents of Loma Linda, California, lived a decade or more longer on average than other Californians. Red meat consumption is lower on average in the Adventist community than in the rest of the United States, so researchers did an analysis to determine whether the trends in meat consumption related to mortality also exist in a population with a low meat consumption. The published findings suggested a moderately increased risk of death from all causes, including heart disease, associated with eating even small amounts of processed and unprocessed red meat.

What effect do plant-based diets have on cholesterol levels? Researchers at the Harvard School of Public Health compiled studies that looked at the effects of replacing red meat with a variety of other foods in almost two thousand individuals. The findings showed that diets that included more high-quality plant protein (such as legumes, soy products, and nuts) resulted in lower levels of both total and LDL cholesterol compared to diets with red meat. Adopting a plant-based diet to lower your LDL cholesterol is a good choice whether or not you have elevated Lp(a).

The Portfolio Diet, an eating plan to lower cholesterol, was developed and tested by David Jenkins, MD, of the University of Toronto. This experiment measured the cholesterol metabolism in individuals on a low-carbohydrate diet high in vegetable proteins (such as gluten, soy products, and nuts), fruits, vegetables, cereals, and vegetable oils compared with a high-carbohydrate diet based on low-fat dairy and whole-grain products. For four weeks at a time, forty-seven men and women with high cholesterol consumed one of these diets. Overall, weight loss was similar for both diets, but reductions in LDL cholesterol and particles that carry cholesterol were greater for the low-carbohydrate diet. Reductions in blood pressure were also seen. The authors noted that a low-carbohydrate plant-based diet has lipid-lowering advantages over a high-carbohydrate, low-fat weight-loss diet and may be better for reducing the risk of cardiac disease. While Lp(a) was not studied, lowering cholesterol with a plant-based diet is prudent for anyone with high Lp(a) levels.

The massive Global Burden of Disease Study reported on dietary factors associated with death worldwide. The study indicated that 22 percent of deaths around the world (an estimated eleven million deaths per year) are due to diet choices. Excess meat and processed-meat consumption were listed among the top fifteen dietary factors increasing the risk of death. The consumption of meat was actually a less powerful predictor of death than not eating an adequate amount of whole grains, fruits, nuts, seeds, and vegetables, so this study took a different slant on the protective nature of plant-based foods.

Further health consequences of eating animal-derived foods, along with new insights into why a meat-based diet promotes disease, have been highlighted in a series of recent investigations. Since 1984, a group of more than 2,500 men have been studied in Finland for the development of heart disease. Diets high in animal-based foods and higher meat intake overall were associated with increased mortality. This was especially true among people with a history of type 2 diabetes, cardiovascular disease, or cancer.

What about the effect of diet on the risk for colorectal cancer? A UK study carried out between 2006 and 2010 looked at almost half a million individuals who filled out diet questionnaires. Participants who reported consuming an average of 76 grams of red and processed meat a day had a 20 percent higher risk of colorectal cancer than people who ate only 21 grams per day. Participants who had the highest intake of fiber (in this case from bread and breakfast cereals) had a 14 percent lower risk of colorectal cancer than those eating little fiber.

One of the most popular dietary trends in the past decade has been to ditch grains, legumes, and dairy products in favor of a diet structured more closely to the supposed Paleolithic diet of thousands of years ago. In a randomized Australian study of subjects eating a typical local diet versus a Paleo diet, researchers measured TMAO, a substance that is created by ingesting red meat. TMAO has been shown to increase atherosclerosis of blood vessels, increase platelet clumping and clotting, and enhance scarring of kidney and heart tissue. Measurements of TMAO blood levels were higher in people who adopted the Paleo diet, which is heavy in meat, and in people whose fiber intake was low, both of which are concerning.

Although studies have linked the consumption of animal-derived foods in general, and red meat in particular, with heart disease in humans, we are still learning new causes of this risk. One newly discovered route to developing damaged heart arteries was described in detail in a recent animal research study. A compound called Neu5Gc can be found in the blood vessels and other tissues of most animal species—except for humans. We lack the ability to create Neu5Gc, so our bodies fight it as if it were a foreign invader. Red meat is rich in Neu5Gc. In this study, when lab animals with metabolisms similar to humans were fed foods rich in Neu5Gc and fats (such as meat), they developed 2.4 times more atherosclerosis than the animals not fed those foods. Choosing plant-based foods, which are naturally free of Neu5Gc, is a wise choice for all, but particularly for people with elevated Lp(a).

A serious allergy to red meat is advancing across the United States as a result of the spread of a particular type of tick, the lone star tick. People who are bitten by this tick can develop an antibody to a compound called alpha-gal, which is found in red meat. A reaction can occur that may result in hives, wheezing, a runny nose, or even anaphylaxis, a potentially deadly condition. In a study in Virginia, individuals with antibodies to alpha-gal from a tick bite had more heart disease than those without these antibodies. This provides one more reason to avoid meat and the potential for heart disease.

Since those first reports that heart disease can be reversed by intensive lifestyle changes that include a plant-based diet low in added fats, the evidence has become so robust that the Ornish Lifestyle Medicine program was recognized by Medicare in 2010 for reimbursement as a therapy for heart disease. A similar program based out of the Pritikin Longevity Center in southern Florida received the same Medicare designation for intensive therapy and reversal of heart disease with dietary therapy. Adopting a lifestyle that reverses heart disease works for even the sickest patients worldwide and is the recommended diet and lifestyle for patients who inherit elevated Lp(a) to minimize their risk of future heart disease.

Eating for Cardiovascular Health

The take-away message from all of these studies is that making small changes to diets that contain animal-based foods will not be nearly as successful at reducing the risk of heart disease, arterial blockages, and high cholesterol, blood pressure, and blood glucose levels as changing to a diet that features only plant-based foods. We also know that anything someone with high Lp(a) levels does to improve overall heart and vascular health will be protective, even though these practices may not actually lower their Lp(a).

We can look at the individual components of plant-based foods that are most protective, such as fiber and antioxidants, but simply adding fiber and antioxidant supplements will not confer the same protections as the whole foods themselves. All the nutrients in plant-based foods work in concert with each other to increase overall nutrient absorption and improve how the body utilizes them.

The recipes in this book will provide you with some delicious options you can use to adopt a diet based entirely on plants—the most effective strategy I know of at this time for staving off chronic illness. Start by replacing one of your daily meals with one of these plant-based recipes. Don't be discouraged if it takes several tries to find a recipe that becomes a favorite. Also note that most people rotate among their favorite five to ten meals, so you don't need to master an entire cookbook's worth of recipes to find delicious options that you and your family will want to stick with. Beverly Lynn Bennett is a proven master at developing flavorful plant-based recipes that are easy to prepare. I know you'll get a great start by browsing through her dishes (see pages 33–135).

A Personal Approach to Controlling High Lipoprotein(a)

Currently, no large, long-term studies exist that provide a definitive approach for someone with high Lp(a), and no specific therapy for a high Lp(a) level is generally recommended or agreed upon by medical professionals. The guidelines that do exist emphasize managing lifestyle and LDL cholesterol levels, which are certainly reasonable recommendations. But there is no course of treatment that directly influences the level of Lp(a), not even the few approaches I discussed in chapter 2 that show promise. My strategy is to create a personalized plan for each of my patients.

I embrace the recent recommendation by the European Society of Cardiology that everyone consider obtaining at least one measurement of their Lp(a) level. I have had my Lp(a) level checked, and it is undetectable. However, if my Lp(a) were elevated (say, 180 nmol/L), I would consider the following steps:

1. Although I have no history of cardiovascular disease, I am over sixty years old and at risk due to age and male gender. Therefore, I would have a carotid intima-medial thickness (CIMT) digital ultrasound (available at my preventive center and a handful of other sites around the country) and a coronary artery calcium score (CACS), as described in the SHAPE Society guidelines (see page 9). The results of these tests would determine my risk and "arterial age." (In reality, my CIMT is free of thickening or plaque, and my CACS is zero.)

2. Using a stethoscope, I would determine if any cardiac murmur (abnormal sounds) were present on a physical exam of my heart. If so, I would have an echocardiogram to assess my aortic valve for calcification and stenosis. I would also review the CACS for any evidence of calcification of the aortic valve as well as other structures, such as the aorta, that are seen on the CIMT scan.

3. I would do a thorough panel of advanced labs, including LDL particles, inflammatory and metabolic markers, genetic markers (such as apolipoprotein E, or ApoE), thyroid hormones, and levels of vitamins D and B_{12}, folate, and omega-3. If there were any suggestion of a low-testosterone syndrome (such as reduced muscle mass, erectile dysfunction, and depression), I would check hormone levels. In a perimenopausal woman, I would check the appropriate hormone levels too.

4. I would review my diet, level of fitness, stress levels, sleep schedule, smoking history, family history (my father had early coronary artery disease), blood pressure, social connections, relationships, and support groups. Having an active and supportive social life has been shown to lower stress and contribute to health and longevity.

5. After evaluating my diet (plant-based for over forty years), I would review the evidence for a whole-foods plant-based diet (as studied by Dean Ornish, MD; Caldwell Esselstyn, MD; and other physicians) to prevent and reverse atherosclerotic disease, prostate disease, and aging, and I would adopt a diet free of animal products and most or all added oils. In view of recent data showing that Lp(a) may decline on a whole-foods plant-based diet, I would feel confident that this was the dietary plan that would most favor my long-term freedom from heart disease and stroke.

6. If I wasn't already exercising, I would search for a program I could follow consistently. I would strive for the goal of 150 minutes a week (about twenty-two minutes a day) of moderate exercise that the American Heart Association recommends. My goal would be a workout intense enough to produce some sweat but with the lowest risk of injury. I would rotate a few stretching routines, such as yoga, with some lightweight lifting and cardio routines using high-intensity interval training to maximize my gains. If I had physical limitations, I would be satisfied with a brisk walk outside or on a treadmill as often as possible. Any exercise is better than none.

7. If my CACS was over 100 or my CIMT showed significant plaque, I would add an 81 mg aspirin daily, unless I had a history of significant bleeding.

8. I would maximize my intake of vitamin C and lysine in response to the theory put forth by two-time Nobel Prize winner Linus Pauling, PhD, and the animal research of his student Matthias Rath, MD, that these essential elements will protect the health of my arteries. I would begin

by increasing my intake of foods rich in these nutrients, such as citrus, leafy greens, and legumes. There are inexpensive supplements that combine vitamin C and lysine in powders and capsules, and the toxicity of these supplements is very low. I would strive to add at least 1,500 mg of vitamin C and 1,500 mg of lysine dissolved in water twice a day. Lp(a) levels are not expected to drop with the use of these nutrients, so there is no way to directly assess their value beyond the theory that they'll protect my arteries, but the goal here is to do everything I can to maximize heart health.

9. I would add L-carnitine (500 mg twice a day) and CoQ10 (200 mg per day), as both can safely lower Lp(a) and are relatively inexpensive. I would check my TMAO blood level (see pages 16–17) and get a repeat test of my Lp(a) level at a Quest lab six to eight weeks after starting L-carnitine. If the level was significantly elevated, I would consider stopping L-carnitine, as it may promote the formation of TMAO, which may promote atherosclerosis. However, on a whole-foods plant-based diet, the TMAO level could be expected to be normal, even with L-carnitine supplementation. If these agents did not lower my Lp(a) level in two to three months, I would consider stopping them.

10. The final point would be managing my cholesterol. If I had a significantly elevated LDL cholesterol or LDL particle number, I would adopt a whole-foods plant-based diet and an exercise program, and I would recheck these values in eight weeks. As this diet is free of cholesterol and low in or free of saturated fat, some people who absorb cholesterol more efficiently than most (called "hyperabsorbers") respond dramatically, with a 100 mg/dl drop in total cholesterol in a short time, particularly if they are coming off of a standard Western diet. If my LDL cholesterol did not decrease to well under 100 mg/dl, I would consider what my CACS report indicated. If it was zero or close to zero, I might hold off taking a statin and wait a few more months to determine what effects diet, L-carnitine, and CoQ10 produced on repeat testing. If my calcium score was elevated (particularly if it was over 100) and my LDL cholesterol was elevated in spite of my lifestyle changes, I would consider taking a statin medication most or all days of the week and reassess my LDL cholesterol levels in eight weeks. I would be certain I had 200 mg a day of CoQ10 in my supplement plan if I were on a statin because statins can inhibit the production of CoQ10.

If my cholesterol test showed a low LDL cholesterol level, or if my LDL responded to lifestyle measures, I would not rush to add a statin. Niacin as a stand-alone therapy is still incorporated into some current reviews and guidelines. Niacin has the potential to lower LDL cholesterol and triglyceride levels, raise HDL cholesterol (which may or may not be beneficial), and lower Lp(a). I would use extended-release niacin and start at 500 mg twice a day. I would take an 81 mg aspirin about thirty minutes before taking niacin, or I would take it with unsweetened apple-sauce if flushing were a significant issue.

I have treated many patients with niacin and seen major reductions in Lp(a) levels. The amount of the drop in Lp(a) levels is unpredictable, though, and the reduction may range from 25 to 80 percent. I have also seen intolerable flushing, liver enzyme elevations, and rare rashes. I have not seen any significant blood sugar issues, fever, infections, or muscle weakness. The decision to use niacin must be the result of a discussion of the pros and cons with the patient. I do not use niacin and statins simultaneously.

Ezetimibe is a well-tolerated medication that is not a statin. It has shown the potential to reduce adverse events such as heart attacks when used with a statin or when used alone. I would take it in addition to a statin if I did not reach low levels of LDL cholesterol with a plant-based diet or with a statin alone. I'd use it alone if a statin created intolerable side effects, such as muscle aches. I would consider taking it with niacin if statins were not tolerated and LDL cholesterol levels on niacin alone did not reach the desired levels.

If my LDL cholesterol was very high and did not respond to diet and a statin (with or without ezetimibe), or if I could not tolerate a statin (usually because of muscle aches), I would apply for a PCSK9 inhibitor. I would use this alone at first, but I might combine it with a statin and even with ezetimibe, too, if needed to reach LDL cholesterol goals. In the future, I would consider an ASO (see page 19) when FDA approval was completed and adequate assessments of its efficacy and safety were established.

BEVERAGES AND BREAKFASTS

5

melon, mango, and green tea SMOOTHIE

Eating more fresh melon, such as cantaloupe and honeydew, can be quite beneficial, as its low-sodium and high-potassium content can help regulate blood pressure levels and reduce the risk of heart attack. Use your favorite type of melon to make this smoothie. It will quench your thirst while giving you an energizing boost from the caffeine in the green tea.

1½ cups cubed **melon** (such as cantaloupe, crenshaw, or honeydew)

1 cup cubed **mango**

1 cup **baby spinach** or other stemmed leafy greens, lightly packed

1 cup cold **green tea**, or 1 cup cold water and 1 teaspoon matcha green tea powder

1 stalk **celery**, sliced

¼ cup **raw almonds** or **walnuts**

1 teaspoon **chia seeds**

½ teaspoon **ground turmeric**

1 Put all the ingredients in a blender and process until smooth.

2 Scrape down the blender jar with a silicone spatula and process for 15 seconds longer. Serve immediately.

cherry cobbler green SMOOTHIE

Makes 1 serving

A high-fiber diet can help reduce the risk of obesity, diabetes, and heart disease. Rolled oats, which are rich in soluble fiber, are commonly served by the bowlful for breakfast, but they're also great for thickening smoothies and boosting their fiber content. Although this creamy smoothie contains iron-rich greens along with rolled oats, it tastes surprisingly like a cherry cobbler.

1 cup fresh or frozen pitted sweet or sour **cherries**

1 **banana**, broken into 3 pieces

1 cup stemmed and coarsely chopped **kale, power greens,** or other **leafy greens,** lightly packed

½ cup plain **oat yogurt** or other **nondairy yogurt**

½ cup **water** or **coconut water**

2 tablespoons **old-fashioned rolled oats**

1 tablespoon **brown sugar,** or 2 pitted soft **dates**

1 piece (½ inch) **fresh ginger,** coarsely chopped

1½ teaspoons **maca powder**

1½ teaspoons **whole flaxseeds,** or 1 teaspoon **chia seeds**

½ teaspoon **ground cinnamon**

½ teaspoon **vanilla extract**

1 Put all the ingredients in a blender and process until smooth.

2 Scrape down the blender jar with a silicone spatula and process for 15 seconds longer. Serve immediately.

Variation **PEACH COBBLER GREEN SMOOTHIE** Replace the cherries with 1 cup frozen sliced peaches or 1 fresh peach, sliced.

get-you-going psyllium SMOOTHIE BOWL

Makes 1 serving

When psyllium husks are mixed with liquid, they thicken into a gel, which is why the husks are commonly used as a fiber supplement. A daily dose of psyllium can also help lower LDL levels. One of the easiest and tastiest ways to add psyllium to your diet is this stunning fuchsia-pink smoothie bowl that will help "get you going" in multiple ways!

½ cup fresh or frozen **berries** (such as blackberries, blueberries, raspberries, or strawberries)

½ cup halved seedless **red or green grapes**

½ cup plain **oat milk** or other **nondairy milk**

½ **avocado**, diced

¼ cup diced **beet** or **carrot**

2 pitted **soft prunes**, or 1 pitted **soft date**

1½ teaspoons **hemp seeds**

1½ teaspoons **psyllium husk powder**

½ cup diced or sliced **fruit**, ⅓ cup fresh **berries**, or 2 tablespoons **pomegranate arils**

2 tablespoons whole or diced **dried fruit** (such as blueberries, cherries, cranberries, dates, figs, goji berries, mulberries, or raisins)

2 tablespoons coarsely chopped **raw nuts**, or 1 tablespoon **raw seeds**

1. Put the berries, grapes, milk, avocado, beet, prunes, and hemp seeds in a blender and process until smooth.

2. Scrape down the blender jar with a silicone spatula. Add the psyllium husk powder and process for 30 seconds longer. The mixture should be very thick, with a consistency similar to soft-serve ice cream.

3. Transfer to a bowl and top with the fresh fruit, dried fruit, and nuts. Serve immediately.

TIP

Psyllium, which comes from the seeds of the herb *Plantago ovata*, can be purchased as either whole or powdered seeds, or as whole or powdered husks, and can be found at most major retailers and natural food stores. Use only pure psyllium husk powder to prepare the recipes in this book.

red, black, and blue fruit salad WITH CHILE-LIME DRESSING

Makes 4 servings

Looking for ways to lower your blood pressure? Eat more watermelon! It's an excellent source of the amino acid L-citrulline, which may help regulate blood pressure levels and reduce the risk of hypertension. Watermelon pairs nicely with fresh berries and grapes in this refreshing, colorful fruit salad. The mildly spicy dressing gives it a bit of a kick.

Juice of 1 **lime** (2 tablespoons)

1 tablespoon **agave nectar**

½ teaspoon **chili powder, ancho chile powder,** or **chipotle chile powder**

2 cups cubed seedless **watermelon**

1 cup halved seedless **red grapes**

1 cup fresh **blackberries**

1 cup fresh **blueberries**

1 cup hulled and thinly sliced fresh **strawberries**

1 To make the dressing, put the lime juice, agave nectar, and chili powder in a small bowl and stir to combine.

2 To make the fruit salad, put the watermelon, grapes, blackberries, blueberries, and strawberries in a large bowl. Pour the dressing over the top and gently stir to combine. Serve immediately.

Save for Later Stored in an airtight container, the fruit salad will keep for 3 days in the refrigerator.

TIP Leftovers can be processed in a blender for a quick smoothie.

maple and cinnamon overnight oats WITH FRESH FRUIT

Makes 1 serving

Rolled oats and their beneficial bran layer are excellent sources of beta-glucan, a type of soluble fiber that dissolves in water and has been shown to help lower blood cholesterol levels. Prep these oats the night before, and they'll be ready and waiting when you're hungry for breakfast. With plenty of add-in options, you'll never get bored with this bowl of oats.

OATMEAL BASE

½ cup old-fashioned **rolled oats**

½ cup plain **oat milk** or other **nondairy milk**

1 tablespoon **maple syrup**

1 teaspoon **ground flaxseeds** or **flaxseed meal**

½ teaspoon **ground cinnamon**

½ teaspoon **vanilla extract** (optional)

TOPPINGS

½ cup diced or sliced **fresh fruit** (such as apples, bananas, berries, mangoes, peaches, pears, pomegranate arils, or a combination)

2 tablespoons whole or diced **dried fruit** (such as apricots, cranberries, dates, figs, goji berries, or raisins)

2 tablespoons coarsely chopped **raw nuts** (such as almonds, pecans, or walnuts), or 1 tablespoon **hemp seeds**

1 To make the oatmeal base, put the oats, milk, maple syrup, flaxseeds, cinnamon, and optional vanilla extract in a small bowl or a 14-ounce glass jar and stir to combine. Cover and refrigerate for 8 to 12 hours.

2 Stir well, then top with the fresh fruit, dried fruit, and nuts. Serve immediately.

Variation

> **CARROT CAKE OVERNIGHT OATS** Replace the diced fresh fruit with ½ cup grated carrots. For the dried fruit and nuts, use 2 tablespoons raisins and 2 tablespoons chopped walnuts, and add 1 tablespoon unsweetened shredded dried coconut.

TIP

> Feel free to prepare more than one serving of overnight oats at a time. Stored in individual airtight containers in the refrigerator (without the toppings), the oats will keep for 5 days. Add the toppings just before serving.

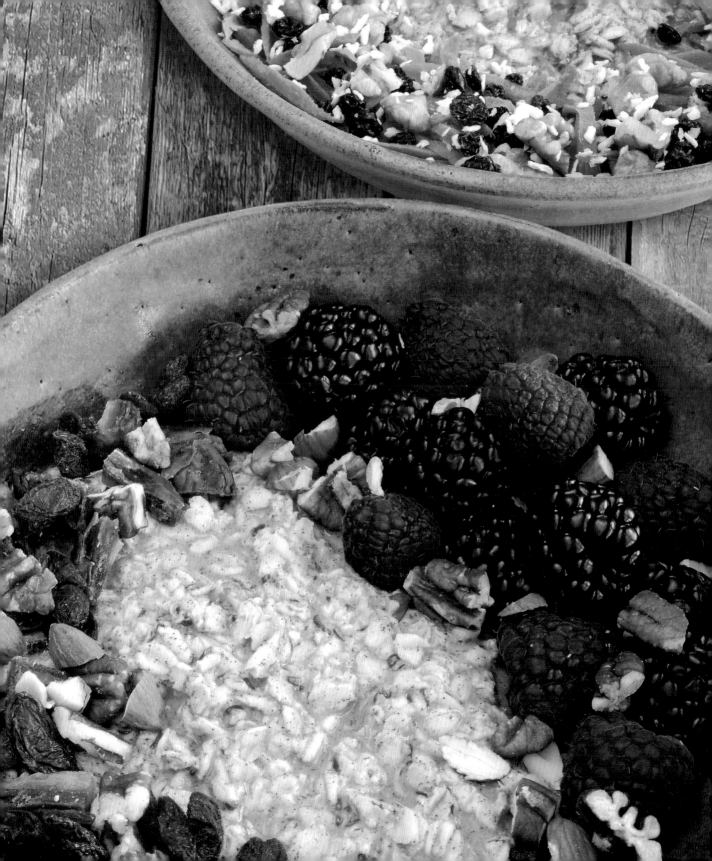

buckwheat and chia seed porridge WITH STRAWBERRY-RHUBARB COMPOTE

Makes 1 serving

Oats aren't the only food that can be soaked overnight to make a tasty bowl of porridge. The base of this cold and creamy breakfast bowl is made with soaked buckwheat groats and chia seeds. As buckwheat is related to rhubarb, it seems only fitting to pair it with a strawberry and rhubarb compote, which is sweetened with a bit of agave nectar and orange juice. The compote can also be prepped ahead and makes enough for several servings.

STRAWBERRY-RHUBARB COMPOTE (makes 1⅓ cups)

1¼ cups sliced **strawberries**

1 cup sliced (1-inch pieces) fresh **rhubarb**

Juice of 1 **orange** (⅓ to ½ cup)

2 tablespoons **water**

2 tablespoons **agave nectar** or **maple syrup**

PORRIDGE BASE

2 cups **water**

½ cup **buckwheat groats**, rinsed

⅓ cup plain **almond milk** or other **nondairy milk**

1 tablespoon **agave nectar** or **maple syrup**

1 tablespoon **unsweetened shredded dried coconut** (optional)

1½ teaspoons **chia seeds**

½ teaspoon **vanilla extract**

Pinch **sea salt**

1 To make the compote, put all the ingredients in a small saucepan and stir to combine. Bring to a boil over high heat. Decrease the heat to low and simmer, stirring occasionally, until the fruit is soft, 20 to 25 minutes. Serve warm or cold.

2 To make the porridge base, combine the water and buckwheat groats in a small bowl. Cover and refrigerate for 8 to 12 hours.

3 Drain the buckwheat groats in a fine-mesh strainer, rinse with cold water, and drain again. Transfer to a food processor and pulse several times until coarsely chopped. Scrape down the work bowl with a silicone spatula.

4 Add the milk, agave nectar, optional coconut, chia seeds, vanilla extract, and salt and process until smooth and creamy. Transfer to a small bowl. Top with ⅓ cup of the compote. Serve immediately.

Variation

For a totally raw version, omit the compote and top each serving with ⅓ cup sliced strawberries and ½ banana, sliced.

Save for Later

Stored in an airtight container in the refrigerator, the compote will keep for 5 days.

avocado toast WITH TOMATO AND ALMOND-HEMP PARMESAN

Makes 2 slices, 1 serving

A recent study found that the monounsaturated fats in avocados help to decrease LDL and overall cholesterol levels, leading some researchers to recommend eating one avocado a day to potentially reduce the risk of heart disease. For the best flavor, make sure the avocado is fully ripe before eating it or using it in recipes. It's essential to use a fully ripened one for avocado toast.

1 **avocado**, diced

Juice of ½ **lemon** (2 tablespoons)

Sea salt

Crushed **red pepper flakes**

2 slices **whole-grain bread**, toasted, or 2 **rice cakes**

1 **Roma tomato**, diced

Balsamic vinegar or **Balsamic Vinegar Reduction** (see page 77; optional)

1 to 2 tablespoons **Almond-Hemp Parmesan** (page 50)

1 Put the avocado and lemon juice in a small bowl and mash with a fork until as smooth and creamy as desired. Season with salt and red pepper flakes to taste.

2 Spread the avocado mixture on the toasted bread. Top with the diced tomato and drizzle with a little balsamic vinegar if desired. Sprinkle the Parmesan over the top.

Variation

AVOCADO PESTO TOAST Replace the avocado mixture with ½ cup Avocado, Spinach, and Hemp Seed Pesto (page 51).

Variation

POMEGRANATE AVOCADO TOAST Omit the diced tomato and optional balsamic vinegar. Top each piece of avocado toast with 2 tablespoons pomegranate arils and sprinkle with the Parmesan.

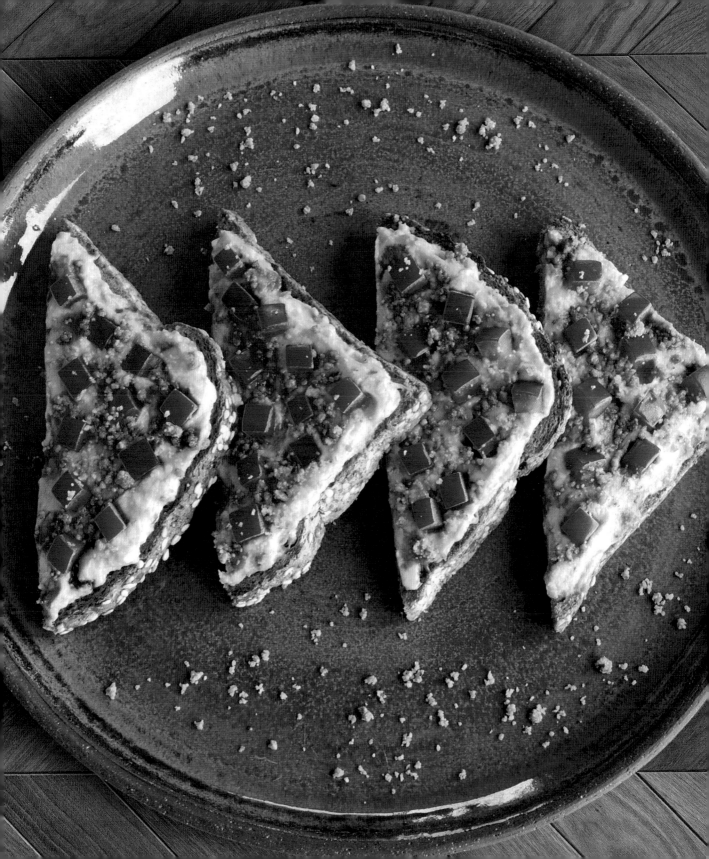

apple-seed OATCAKES

Makes 8 pancakes, 4 servings

It's said that an apple a day keeps the doctor away. Surely, then, combining apples with oats and omega–3 rich chia, hemp, and flaxseeds all in one bite must help keep the heart doctor away! Well, maybe not if your doctor is Joel Kahn, America's Healthy Heart Doc, as he surely would give you a prescription to make a batch of these wholesome pancakes. Serve them with your favorite toppings, such as maple syrup, agave nectar, nut butter, vegan yogurt, jam, or jelly.

1½ cups **oat flour** (see page 45)

1 tablespoon **chia seeds**

1 tablespoon **hemp seeds**

1 tablespoon **ground flaxseeds** or **flaxseed meal**

1 teaspoon **baking powder**

½ teaspoon **baking soda**

½ teaspoon **sea salt**

1½ cups plain **oat milk, soy milk,** or **almond milk**

¼ cup plain **oat yogurt** or other **nondairy yogurt**

2 tablespoons **maple syrup** or **agave nectar**

1 tablespoon **cider vinegar**

1 teaspoon **vanilla extract**

1 cup coarsely grated **apple,** lightly packed

1 Put the oat flour, chia seeds, hemp seeds, flaxseeds, baking powder, baking soda, and salt in a large bowl and whisk to combine.

2 Add the milk, yogurt, maple syrup, vinegar, and vanilla extract and whisk until just combined. A few lumps are fine; don't overmix or the pancakes will be tough. Gently stir in the apple. Let the batter rest for 5 minutes to allow it to thicken slightly.

3 Lightly mist a large nonstick skillet or griddle with cooking spray. Heat over medium heat.

4 When the skillet is hot, portion the batter into it using ⅓ cup of batter for each pancake. Cook until the edges of the pancakes are dry and the bottoms are lightly browned, 3 to 4 minutes. Flip the pancakes over and cook until lightly browned on the other side, 2 to 3 minutes.

5 Lightly mist the skillet with cooking spray between batches as needed and repeat with the remaining batter. Serve hot.

Variation

> **APPLE-SEED BUCKWHEAT PANCAKES** Replace all or half of the oat flour with buckwheat flour and add an additional 2 tablespoons oat milk.

Variation

> Replace the grated apple with 1 cup chopped fresh fruit or fresh or frozen berries.

Save for Later

> Stored in an airtight container, the pancakes will keep for 3 days in the refrigerator.

TIP

> **HOMEMADE OAT FLOUR** To make oat flour, put rolled oats in a blender or food processor and process into a fine powder, 1 to 2 minutes. One cup of rolled oats will yield approximately 1 cup of oat flour. Oat flour can often be used measure for measure to replace all-purpose or other wheat-based flour. It can also be used as a gluten-free replacement for wheat flour in many recipes.

southwestern tofu SCRAMBLE

You can lower your LDL cholesterol easily by giving up eggs, both for breakfast and for good. For decades, tofu has been used as a cholesterol-free stand-in for eggs, especially for making heart-healthy tofu scrambles, much like this Southwestern-inspired one with its colorful blend of peppers, beans, and cilantro. If you like, top it with your favorite hot sauce or salsa (or both), or turn it into a breakfast burrito by rolling it up in a tortilla with sliced avocado.

1 pound firm or extra-firm **tofu**

⅓ cup low-sodium **vegetable broth** or **water**

2 tablespoons **nutritional yeast flakes**

1 tablespoon reduced-sodium **tamari**

1 teaspoon **chili powder**

½ teaspoon **garlic granules**

½ teaspoon **ground turmeric**

½ teaspoon **smoked paprika**

¼ teaspoon freshly ground **black pepper**

⅓ cup diced **green bell pepper**

⅓ cup diced **red bell pepper**

1 **jalapeño chile**, cut in half, seeded, and finely diced

⅔ cup cooked **beans** (such as black, kidney, or red)

⅓ cup thinly sliced **green onions**

⅓ cup chopped **fresh cilantro** or **parsley**, lightly packed

1 Using your fingers, crumble the tofu into a large nonstick skillet. Add half of the broth and all of the nutritional yeast, tamari, chili powder, garlic granules, turmeric, paprika, and black pepper. Cook over medium-high heat, stirring occasionally, for 3 minutes.

2 Add the remaining broth and the green bell pepper, red bell pepper, and chile and cook, stirring occasionally, for 5 minutes.

3 Add the beans, green onions, and cilantro and cook, stirring occasionally, for 2 minutes. Serve hot.

Save for Later | Stored in an airtight container, the tofu scramble will keep for 3 days in the refrigerator.

CONDIMENTS, SAUCES, AND SNACKS

6

mango-pineapple SALSA

*I*f you need to up your potassium levels, eat more tropical fruits, such as bananas, mangoes, and pineapples. This sweet and slightly spicy salsa can help you do that quite readily. Serve it with your favorite tortilla chips or spoon it over burritos, salads, or cooked black beans.

2 **mangoes,** diced

¾ cup diced **red bell pepper**

½ cup canned **pineapple tidbits,** drained

½ cup diced **red onion**

¼ cup chopped **fresh cilantro,** lightly packed

1 **jalapeño chile,** seeded and finely diced

1 tablespoon minced **garlic**

Juice of 1 **lime** (2 tablespoons)

Sea salt

Freshly ground **black pepper**

1 Put the mangoes, bell pepper, pineapple, onion, cilantro, chile, garlic, and lime juice in a medium bowl and stir to combine.

2 Season with salt and pepper to taste. Serve immediately.

Variation **MANGO-PAPAYA SALSA** Use only 1 mango, omit the pineapple, and add 1 cup diced papaya.

Save for Later Stored in an airtight container, the salsa will keep for 3 days in the refrigerator.

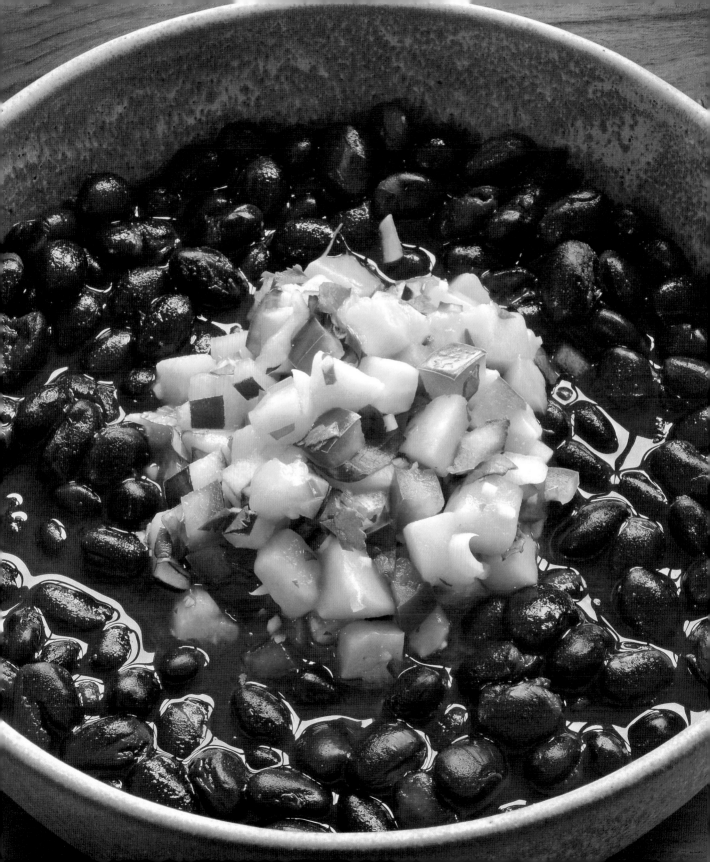

almond-hemp **PARMESAN**

his plant-based alternative to Parmesan cheese has a slightly salty, cheesy flavor that is surprisingly similar to its dairy-based counterpart. This vegan version, however, is cholesterol-free and also supplies vitamin B_{12} and omega-3 fatty acids, thanks to the nutritional yeast, almonds, and hemp seeds it contains.

⅓ cup **raw sliced almonds** or **blanched slivered almonds,** or ½ cup **almond flour**

⅓ cup **hemp seeds**

⅓ cup **nutritional yeast flakes**

½ teaspoon **sea salt**

¼ teaspoon **onion powder**

¼ teaspoon **garlic granules**

1 Put all the ingredients in a food processor and process for 1 minute.

2 Scrape down the work bowl with a silicone spatula and process until finely ground, 30 to 60 seconds.

Save for Later Stored in an airtight container, the Parmesan will keep for 1 month in the refrigerator.

avocado, spinach, and hemp seed PESTO

I t's easy to make delicious pesto without any oil or dairy. The combination of avocado, hemp seeds, and nutritional yeast in this lighter version mimics the creamy texture and cheesy flavor of traditional pesto. Keep this pesto on hand to flavor sauces or soups, use as a spread for toast or sandwiches, or toss with cooked pasta or zucchini noodles (zoodles) for a tasty meal.

1 cup **baby spinach,** lightly packed

1 cup **fresh basil leaves,** lightly packed

½ **avocado,** diced

¼ cup **hemp seeds,** or 2 tablespoons hemp seeds and 2 tablespoons walnuts

2 tablespoons **nutritional yeast flakes** or **Almond-Hemp Parmesan** (page 45)

Juice of ½ **lemon** (2 tablespoons)

2 large cloves **garlic**

¼ teaspoon crushed **red pepper flakes** (optional)

Sea salt

Freshly ground **black pepper** or **white pepper**

1 Put the spinach, basil, avocado, hemp seeds, nutritional yeast, lemon juice, garlic, and optional red pepper flakes in a food processor and process until smooth, 1 to 2 minutes. Season with salt and pepper to taste.

2 Scrape down the work bowl with a silicone spatula and process for 15 seconds longer.

Save for Later   Stored in an airtight container, the pesto will keep for 3 days in the refrigerator.

OIL-FREE roasted chickpeas

Makes 1 cup, 4 servings

Looking for a tasty, fiber-filled snack? Chickpeas to the rescue! Snack on these seasoned, oven-roasted morsels by the handful, if you like, as they're oil-free. You can also use them as a topping for salads, pasta, or grain dishes.

1 can (15 ounces) **chickpeas, drained** (reserve liquid for aquafaba)

1 tablespoon **aquafaba** (see page 53)

1½ teaspoons reduced-sodium **tamari,** or ½ teaspoon **sea salt**

1½ teaspoons **nutritional yeast flakes**

½ teaspoon **garlic granules**

½ teaspoon **onion powder**

½ teaspoon **paprika**

1 Put the chickpeas on a clean kitchen towel or on paper towels and let air-dry for 10 minutes.

2 Preheat the oven to 375 degrees F. Line a baking sheet with parchment paper or a silicone baking mat.

3 Transfer the chickpeas to the lined baking sheet and spread into a single layer. Bake for 30 minutes, shaking the pan every 15 minutes to ensure even baking. Remove from the oven.

4 Put the aquafaba, tamari, nutritional yeast, garlic granules, onion powder, and paprika in a small bowl and stir to combine. Add the chickpeas and stir until evenly coated.

5 Transfer the chickpeas back to the lined baking sheet and spread into a single layer. Bake for 10 to 15 minutes, until the chickpeas are golden brown, dry, and slightly crunchy.

6 Turn off the oven and leave the oven door partially open. Let the chickpeas cool completely in the oven, as this will make them drier and crispier.

Save for Later

Stored in an airtight container, the roasted chickpeas will keep for 5 days at room temperature.

Tip

VERSATILE AQUAFABA Have you heard about aquafaba? It's the liquid from drained cooked or canned chickpeas that is often discarded. Aquafaba has taken the culinary world by storm because of its incredible ability to replace eggs in a variety of recipes. Due to its high-protein content, aquafaba can be used as a binder; but even more miraculously, it can be whipped to create a light and fluffy foam that resembles beaten egg whites!

To drain chickpeas and reserve the aquafaba, put a fine-mesh strainer over a bowl and pour the chickpeas into the strainer. Transfer the aquafaba from the bowl to an airtight container and store in the refrigerator for up to 1 week.

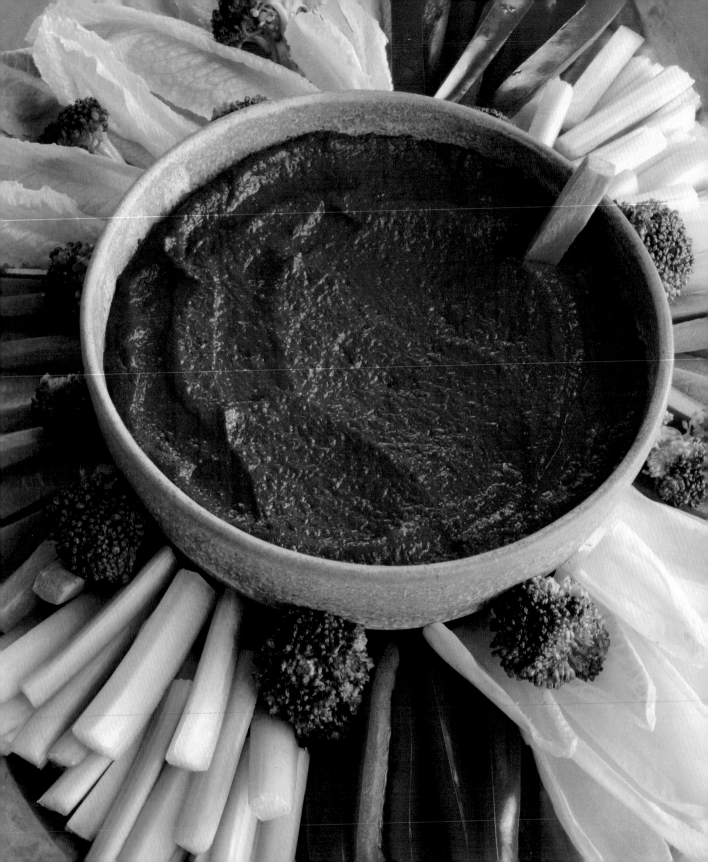

beet HUMMUS

Beets contain dietary nitrates that can be converted into nitric oxide, which can cause blood vessels to dilate and blood pressure to drop. This is a good thing, as it can reduce the risk of heart attack and stroke. If you love beets, then you've gotta try this vibrantly colored hummus. Serve it with sliced fresh veggies, pita bread, or crackers. Its flavor can't be beat!

1 small **beet** (baseball-sized or about 6 ounces)

3 large cloves **garlic**

1 can (15 ounces) **chickpeas, drained** (reserve liquid for aquafaba)

3 tablespoons **tahini**

Juice of ½ **lemon** (2 tablespoons)

2 tablespoons **aquafaba** (see page 53) or **water**

½ teaspoon **ground cumin**

½ teaspoon **sea salt**

1 To roast the beet, preheat the oven to 425 degrees F. Wrap the beet in foil, and put it in a pie pan or other baking pan. Bake for 45 to 55 minutes, until the beet is tender and easily pierced with a knife. Remove from the oven. Let cool for 10 minutes.

2 When the beet is cool, carefully peel it using a knife and cut it into small pieces. Transfer to a food processor. Add the garlic and process until the beet is finely chopped.

3 Add the chickpeas, tahini, lemon juice, aquafaba, cumin, and salt and process until smooth. Scrape down the work bowl with a silicone spatula and process for 15 seconds longer.

Save for Later | Stored in an airtight container, the hummus will keep for 5 days in the refrigerator.

TIP | It's a good idea to roast more than one beet, as roasted beets are delicious. They can be cubed or sliced as desired for use in salads, grain dishes, soups, or smoothies.

creamy cauliflower CHEESE SAUCE

Cauliflower is an excellent source of choline, a nutrient that can help suppress inflammation and prevent cholesterol from accumulating in the liver. Cooked cauliflower is often covered in a cheesy-tasting sauce to make it more appetizing for finicky eaters. Surprisingly, it can also be used as the base of a totally plant-based cheese sauce that can be poured over cooked vegetables, grains, or pasta or used as the saucy component of a casserole.

1½ cups small **white or orange cauliflower** florets

¾ cup **water**

⅓ cup **raw cashews**

¼ cup diced **orange or red bell pepper**

¼ cup diced **shallots** or **yellow onion**

2 large cloves **garlic,** thinly sliced

¼ cup **nutritional yeast flakes**

1 tablespoon **lemon juice**

½ teaspoon **sea salt**

¼ teaspoon **sweet or smoked paprika**

¼ teaspoon **dry mustard**

¼ teaspoon freshly ground **black pepper**

1 Put the cauliflower, water, cashews, bell pepper, shallots, and garlic in a medium saucepan. Bring to a boil over high heat. Cover, decrease the heat to low, and simmer, stirring occasionally, until the cauliflower is soft, 5 to 7 minutes. Remove from the heat. Let cool for 5 minutes.

2 Transfer the vegetables and cooking liquid to a blender. Add the nutritional yeast, lemon juice, salt, paprika, dry mustard, and pepper and process until smooth. Scrape down the blender jar with a silicone spatula and process for 15 seconds longer. Serve hot, warm, or at room temperature.

Variation

CAULIFLOWER QUESO DIP Add ½ cup homemade or store-bought salsa and stir to combine. Can be served as a dip with tortilla chips or vegetables or as a spicy sauce for tacos, burritos, or other dishes.

Save for Later

Stored in an airtight container, the sauce or dip will keep for 5 days in the refrigerator.

quick cashew GRAVY

Makes 2 cups

No roux for you! That's because the famous flour-and-butter combo isn't used in this recipe. Instead, this vegan gravy is thickened with pulverized cashews and chia seeds. Not only is this rich-tasting gravy meat-free, but it also doesn't contain any oil, flour, or soy. Use it to top biscuits, mashed potatoes, baked tofu or tempeh, or other savory dishes.

½ cup **raw cashews**

1½ tablespoons **chia seeds**

1½ cups low-sodium **vegetable broth**

½ cup **white or red wine** (such as Burgundy, Chardonnay, Pinot Noir, or Riesling), or ½ cup additional **vegetable broth**

2 tablespoons **nutritional yeast flakes**

1 teaspoon **garlic granules**

1 teaspoon **onion powder**

½ teaspoon **sea salt**

¼ teaspoon freshly ground **black pepper**

1 Put the cashews and chia seeds in a blender and process until finely ground. Scrape down the blender jar with a silicone spatula.

2 Add the broth, wine, nutritional yeast, garlic granules, onion powder, salt, and pepper and process until smooth.

3 Transfer to a medium saucepan and cook over medium heat, whisking occasionally, until thickened, 3 to 5 minutes. Serve hot.

Save for Later   Stored in an airtight container, the gravy will keep for 5 days in the refrigerator.

SOUPS AND SALADS

7

corn, quinoa, and kidney bean CHILI

Makes 6 cups, 4 servings

Cooking a big pot of chili will fill your home with an irresistible aroma. This fiber-filled version is made with a hearty blend of kidney beans, corn, onions, peppers, and quinoa (for added texture and protein), plus a hint of cacao powder and a generous dose of herbs and spices for great depth of flavor. Serve it by the bowlful, along with your favorite hot sauce, crackers, tortilla chips, or cornbread.

1 cup diced **red or yellow onion**

1 **red or orange bell pepper**, diced

½ **green bell pepper**, diced

1 **serrano or jalapeño chile**, seeded and finely diced

1¾ cups **water** or low-sodium **vegetable broth**

4 large **garlic cloves**, minced

1 tablespoon **cacao powder** or unsweetened cocoa powder

1½ tablespoons **chili powder**

1 teaspoon **dried oregano**

1 teaspoon **ground cumin**

½ teaspoon **ground coriander**

¼ teaspoon **cayenne, ancho chile powder, or chipotle chile powder**

1 can (15 ounces) **kidney beans**, drained and rinsed

1 can (14 ounces) **crushed tomatoes**

1 can (14 ounces) **fire-roasted or regular diced tomatoes**

1 cup fresh or frozen **corn kernels** (do not thaw)

⅓ cup **tricolor quinoa** or other quinoa, rinsed

⅓ cup chopped **fresh cilantro** or **parsley**, lightly packed

Juice of 1 **lime** (2 tablespoons)

Sea salt

Freshly ground **black pepper**

1 Put the onion, red bell pepper, green bell pepper, chile, ¼ cup of the water, and garlic in a large soup pot. Cook over medium-high heat, stirring occasionally, until the water has evaporated, 3 to 5 minutes. Add the cacao powder, chili powder, oregano, cumin, coriander, and cayenne and cook, stirring occasionally, for 1 minute.

2 Add the kidney beans, crushed tomatoes, diced tomatoes, remaining 1½ cups water, corn, and quinoa and stir to combine. Bring to a boil over high heat. Cover, decrease the heat to low, and simmer, stirring occasionally, until the vegetables and quinoa are soft, 20 to 30 minutes.

3 Add the cilantro and lime juice and stir until evenly distributed. Season with salt and pepper to taste. Serve hot.

Variation Replace the kidney beans with other canned beans, such as black, pinto, red, or a combination.

Save for Later Stored in an airtight container, the chili will keep for 5 days in the refrigerator or 2 months in the freezer.

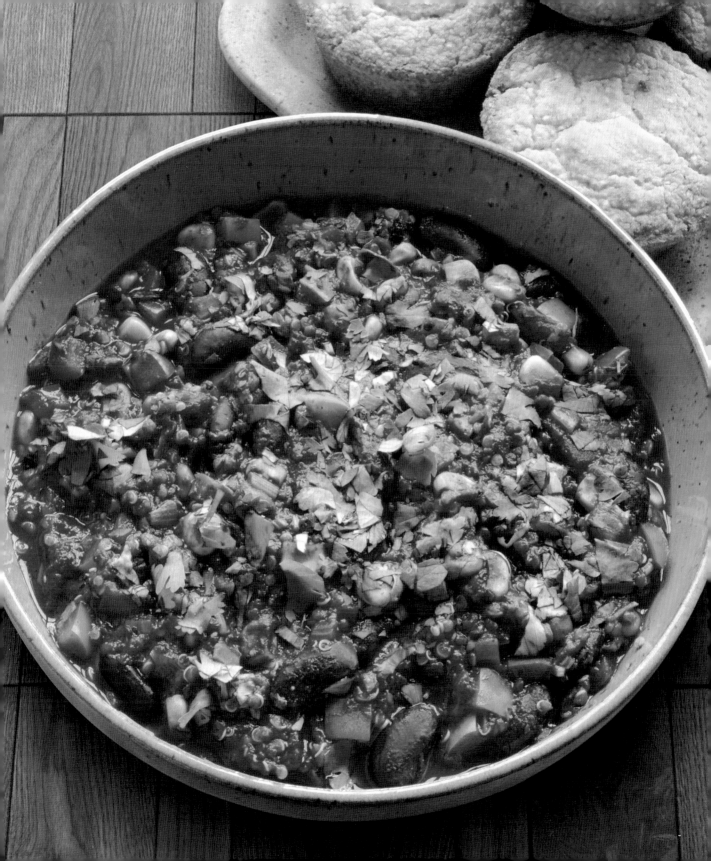

savory tofu, vegetable, and rice SOUP

Makes 6 cups, 4 servings

This is a great soup for when you're feeling a bit under the weather or are just in the mood for some comfort food. The golden broth is made with dried herbs, turmeric, nutritional yeast, and white wine, and this combination elevates the flavor of the humble aromatic vegetables, leafy greens, and rice. As a final flourish, each serving is topped with strips of breaded tofu to create a vegan version of chicken-and-rice soup.

1 **yellow onion,** diced

3 **carrots,** cut in half lengthwise and thinly sliced

2 stalks **celery,** cut in half lengthwise and thinly sliced

4 large cloves **garlic,** minced

4 cups low-sodium **vegetable broth**

½ cup **brown rice, wild rice,** or **mixed-rice blend,** rinsed

1 **bay leaf**

1 tablespoon **Italian seasoning** (or 1 teaspoon each dried basil, oregano, rosemary, and thyme), or 1 tablespoon **poultry seasoning**

1½ teaspoons **dried dill weed**

½ teaspoon freshly ground **black pepper**

2 cups stemmed and coarsely chopped **leafy greens** (such as kale, spinach, or Swiss chard), lightly packed

⅓ cup chopped **fresh parsley,** lightly packed

⅓ cup **white wine** (such as Chardonnay or Riesling)

2 tablespoons **nutritional yeast flakes**

1 tablespoon reduced-sodium **tamari**

¼ teaspoon ground **turmeric** or **curry powder**

4 slices **Oat Bran–Breaded Tofu** or **Tempeh Cutlets** (page 100)

1. Put the onion, carrots, celery, and garlic in a large soup pot. Cover and cook over medium-high heat, stirring occasionally, for 5 minutes.

2. Add the broth, rice, bay leaf, Italian seasoning, dill weed, and pepper and stir to combine. Bring to a boil over high heat. Cover, decrease the heat to low, and simmer, stirring occasionally, until the rice is soft, 30 to 40 minutes.

3. Remove and discard the bay leaf. Add the leafy greens, parsley, wine, nutritional yeast, tamari, and turmeric and stir to combine. Cover and simmer, stirring occasionally, until the greens are tender, 5 to 10 minutes.

4. Remove from the heat. Prior to serving, cut each slice of the breaded tofu or tempeh in half lengthwise, then cut it crosswise into thin strips and place on top of each serving. Serve hot.

Save for Later   Stored in an airtight container, the soup will keep for 3 days in the refrigerator or 2 months in the freezer.

scotch **BROTH**

Makes 7 cups, 5 servings

Barley, like oats, can help lower LDL cholesterol levels, thanks to the beta-glucan fiber it contains. While this soup may be named for the Scots, Scotch broth has been a mainstay meal for centuries throughout most of the United Kingdom. In this vegan version, beer elevates the flavor and stands in for the meat base that is traditionally used.

¼ cup **dried green split peas**, sorted and rinsed

¼ cup **dried yellow split peas**, sorted and rinsed

¼ cup **dried red lentils**, sorted and rinsed

¼ cup **hulled** or **pearl barley**

3 cups low-sodium **vegetable broth**

1 bottle (12 ounces) **beer**

1 small **leek**, cut in half lengthwise and thinly sliced

1 cup peeled and cubed **rutabaga**

1 **parsnip**, peeled and cut into ½-inch cubes

1 **carrot**, cut in half lengthwise and thinly sliced

1 stalk **celery**, cut in half lengthwise and thinly sliced

1 **bay leaf**

2 teaspoons **dried thyme**

2 cups coarsely chopped **savoy cabbage, green cabbage, kale,** or a combination

2 tablespoons **nutritional yeast flakes**

½ teaspoon **sea salt**

¼ teaspoon freshly ground **black pepper**

½ cup chopped **fresh parsley,** lightly packed

1. Put the green split peas, yellow split peas, red lentils, and barley in a fine-mesh strainer and rinse until the water runs clear. Transfer to a large soup pot, cover with water, and let soak for 8 to 12 hours.

2. Drain, rinse, and return the split pea mixture to the large soup pot.

3. Add the broth, beer, leek, rutabaga, parsnip, carrot, celery, bay leaf, and thyme and stir to combine. Bring to a boil over high heat. Cover, decrease the heat to low, and simmer, stirring occasionally, for 1 hour.

4. Remove and discard the bay leaf. Add the cabbage, nutritional yeast, salt, and pepper and stir to combine. Cover and simmer, stirring occasionally, until the split peas are soft, 20 to 30 minutes. Stir in the parsley. Serve hot.

Save for Later

Stored in an airtight container, the soup will keep for 5 days in the refrigerator or 2 months in the freezer.

lentil MINESTRONE

According to research done by David J. A. Jenkins, MD, creator of the Portfolio Diet, eating one cup of beans or lentils every day may help reduce the risk of heart attack and stroke and also help control blood sugar in people with type 2 diabetes. All that aside, legumes are simply delicious, especially in soups like this hearty minestrone, made with earthy lentils, spinach, and your choice of pasta. Use a bean-based pasta to boost your bean intake even more!

6 cups **water**, or 4 cups water and 2 cups **tomato broth**

1¼ cups **dried brown lentils**, sorted and rinsed

1 **yellow onion**, diced

1½ cups peeled and cubed **potatoes** or **turnips**

3 **carrots**, cut in half lengthwise and thinly sliced

2 stalks **celery**, cut in half lengthwise and thinly sliced

1 small **zucchini**, cut into quarters lengthwise and thinly sliced

4 large cloves **garlic**, minced

1½ tablespoons **Italian seasoning** (or 1 teaspoon each dried basil, oregano, rosemary, and thyme)

1 **bay leaf**

8 ounces **spinach** or **lacinato kale**, stemmed and coarsely chopped, or 1 (10-ounce) **package frozen chopped spinach or kale** (do not thaw)

½ cup **whole-grain or bean-based small pasta** (such as ditalini, elbows, orzo, or shells)

⅓ cup **red wine** (such as Burgundy or Pinot Noir), **or 2 tablespoons balsamic or red wine vinegar**

⅓ cup chopped **fresh parsley**, lightly packed

1½ tablespoons **nutritional yeast flakes** or **Almond-Hemp Parmesan** (page 50)

Sea salt

Freshly ground **black pepper**

1. Put the water, lentils, onion, potatoes, carrots, celery, zucchini, garlic, Italian seasoning, and bay leaf in a large soup pot and stir to combine. Bring to a boil over high heat. Cover, decrease the heat to low, and simmer for 30 minutes.

2. Remove and discard the bay leaf. Add the spinach, pasta, and wine and stir to combine. Cover and simmer, stirring occasionally, until the lentils and pasta are soft, 15 to 20 minutes.

3. Add the parsley and nutritional yeast and stir until evenly distributed. Season with salt and pepper to taste. Serve hot.

Variation
Replace the lentils with 1 cup dried cannellini beans or chickpeas, sorted and rinsed. Simmer the soup for an additional 20 to 30 minutes, until the beans are soft.

Save for Later
Stored in an airtight container, the soup will keep for 5 days in the refrigerator or 2 months in the freezer.

tofu chicken salad
WITH APPLES AND GRAPES

Makes 4 cups, 4 servings

When you're craving something sweet and savory, this chicken-free chicken salad will fill the bill. Grapes and apples bring sweetness, and seasoned tofu and crunchy nuts supply the savory. Instead of mayonnaise, lemon juice and yogurt add tang and creaminess. Enjoy this salad on a bed of mixed greens, as a topping for crackers, or as a filling for sandwiches or wraps.

1 pound firm or extra-firm regular **tofu**, pressed (see page 69)

2 tablespoons **nutritional yeast flakes**

1 tablespoon reduced-sodium tamari

½ cup plain **oat yogurt** or other **nondairy yogurt**

1 tablespoon **lemon juice**

1½ teaspoons **chia seeds**

1½ teaspoons **poppy seeds**

½ teaspoon **garlic granules**

½ teaspoon **dried thyme**

½ cup diced **apple**

½ cup halved **seedless red grapes**

⅓ cup coarsely chopped raw or toasted **pecans** or **almonds**

1 stalk **celery**, cut in half lengthwise and thinly sliced

¼ cup finely diced **red onion**

¼ cup chopped **fresh parsley**, lightly packed

Sea salt

Freshly ground **black pepper**

1. Preheat the oven to 400 degrees F. Line a baking sheet with parchment paper or a silicone baking mat.

2. Cut the tofu into 1-inch cubes and put the cubes in a small bowl. Add 1 tablespoon of the nutritional yeast and the tamari. Using your hands, gently toss the cubes until they are evenly coated.

3. Transfer to the lined baking sheet and spread into a single layer, spacing the cubes one-half inch apart. Bake for 30 to 35 minutes, or until golden brown around the edges. Let cool completely on the baking sheet.

4. To make the dressing, put the remaining 1 tablespoon of nutritional yeast and the yogurt, lemon juice, chia seeds, poppy seeds, garlic granules, and thyme in a small bowl and stir to combine.

5 Transfer the tofu to a large bowl. Add the apple, grapes, pecans, celery, onion, and parsley and stir to combine. Add the dressing and gently stir until evenly distributed. Season with salt and pepper to taste. Let sit for 10 minutes to allow the flavors to blend. Serve immediately or thoroughly chilled.

Save for Later

Stored in an airtight container, the tofu chicken salad will keep for 3 days in the refrigerator.

Tip

HOW TO PRESS TOFU Pressing tofu removes excess water, making it denser and meatier. To press it, gently squeeze the block of tofu over the sink to remove any excess water. Take care not to crush the tofu, as the block should remain intact. Put the tofu in a colander in the sink, then put a small plate directly on the tofu. Put a large can or other heavy weight on top of the plate and let the tofu rest and drain for 20 minutes.

niçoise POTATO SALAD

Makes 6 servings

Niçoise salad is an artfully composed classic French dish in which each ingredient is arranged like an edible painting. The salad typically features cooked potatoes, green beans, tomatoes, and olives (as well as some animal products). For this totally plant-based version, these ingredients plus a few more vegetable components are tossed, rather than arranged, for easier preparation of this tangy, upscale potato salad.

SHALLOT-DIJON VINAIGRETTE (makes ¾ cup)

Juice of 1 **lemon** (¼ cup)

¼ cup **white or red wine vinegar**

2 tablespoons finely diced **shallot**

2 tablespoons chopped **fresh tarragon**, or 2 teaspoons **dried tarragon**

1½ tablespoons chopped **fresh dill**, or 1½ teaspoons **dried dill weed**

1½ tablespoons **Dijon mustard** (preferably a whole-grain variety)

1 tablespoon **nutritional yeast flakes**

½ teaspoon **sea salt**

¼ teaspoon freshly ground **black pepper**

POTATO SALAD

6 ounces **fresh green beans** or **purple long beans**, cut into 1½-inch pieces (about 1½ cups)

2 pounds **red-skinned potatoes**, cut into 1-inch cubes, or **small potatoes**, cut into quarters

½ cup halved **cherry tomatoes** or **grape tomatoes**

¼ cup **radishes**, halved and thinly sliced

¼ cup **pitted black olives**, cut in half

¼ cup thinly sliced **green onions**, or 2 tablespoons thinly sliced **chives**

¼ cup chopped **fresh parsley**, lightly packed

1. To make the vinaigrette, put all the ingredients in a small bowl and whisk until well combined. Let sit for at least 10 minutes to allow the flavors to blend.

2. Put a collapsible steamer basket or steamer rack into a large saucepan. Add enough water to just touch the bottom of the collapsible steamer, or make the water two inches deep if using a rack. Cover the saucepan and bring to a boil over medium heat.

3. Steam the green beans until crisp-tender, 4 to 5 minutes. Transfer to a small plate and set aside to cool.

4. Steam the potatoes until just tender and they can be easily pierced with a knife, 10 to 15 minutes. Transfer to a large bowl and let cool for 10 minutes.

5. While the potatoes are still warm, add half of the vinaigrette and stir gently to evenly coat the potatoes. Let the potatoes cool completely.

6. When the potatoes are cool, add the green beans, tomatoes, radishes, olives, green onions, parsley, and the remaining vinaigrette and gently stir to combine. Let sit for 10 minutes to allow the flavors to blend. Serve immediately or thoroughly chilled.

Variation

COMPOSED NIÇOISE POTATO SALAD For a composed salad, keep all of the salad ingredients separate. Arrange a bed of 6 cups of arugula on a large platter. Arrange the coated potatoes, steamed green beans, tomatoes, radishes, olives, and green onions in individual clusters on top of the arugula. Sprinkle the parsley evenly over the salad items, then drizzle the remaining vinaigrette over the top.

Save for Later

Stored in an airtight container, the potato salad will keep for 3 days in the refrigerator.

mediterranean **PASTA SALAD**

The Mediterranean diet is a way of eating based on the traditional cuisine of countries bordering the Mediterranean Sea. This pasta salad is made with Mediterranean-inspired ingredients, such as artichoke hearts, chickpeas, spinach, zucchini, tomatoes, and olives, and is dressed with a tangy vinaigrette. Serve it as is or on a bed of mixed greens or shredded romaine lettuce.

SUN-DRIED TOMATO AND BLACK OLIVE VINAIGRETTE (makes ¾ cup)

4 whole **sun-dried tomatoes,** or ⅓ cup **sun-dried tomato pieces,** lightly packed

3 tablespoons warm **water**

¼ cup **pitted black olives**

2 tablespoons **balsamic vinegar**

2 tablespoons **red wine vinegar**

1 tablespoon **nutritional yeast flakes** or **Almond-Hemp Parmesan** (page 50)

1 tablespoon **spicy brown mustard** or **Dijon mustard**

1 teaspoon **dried basil**

1 teaspoon **dried oregano**

½ teaspoon **paprika**

PASTA SALAD

8 ounces small **whole-grain or bean-based pasta** (such as orzo, penne, rotini, or shells)

1 cup coarsely chopped **baby spinach,** lightly packed

1 cup cooked **chickpeas** or **cannellini beans**

¾ cup thawed frozen or canned (packed in water) **artichoke hearts,** drained and coarsely chopped

¾ cup sliced **zucchini** (cut a small zucchini into quarters lengthwise, then thinly slice)

½ cup halved **cherry tomatoes,** or ⅔ cup **diced tomatoes**

1 stalk **celery,** cut in half lengthwise and thinly sliced

⅓ cup finely diced **red onion**

¼ cup sliced **black or green olives**

¼ cup toasted **pine nuts**

¼ cup chopped **fresh parsley,** lightly packed

Sea salt

Freshly ground **black pepper**

1   To make the vinaigrette, put the sun-dried tomatoes and warm water in a blender and let sit for 10 minutes to allow the tomatoes to rehydrate. Add the olives, balsamic vinegar, wine vinegar, nutritional yeast, mustard, basil, oregano, and paprika and process until smooth. Scrape down the blender jar with a silicone spatula and process for 15 seconds longer. Let the vinaigrette sit for 10 minutes or longer to allow the flavors to blend.

2   Cook the pasta in boiling water according to the package directions. Drain in a colander, rinse under cold water, and drain again. Transfer to a large bowl.

3   Add the spinach, chickpeas, artichoke hearts, zucchini, cherry tomatoes, celery, onion, olives, pine nuts, and parsley and gently stir to combine. Add the vinaigrette and gently toss until evenly distributed. Season with salt and pepper to taste. Let sit for 10 minutes to allow the flavors to blend. Serve immediately or thoroughly chilled.

Variation

MEDITERRANEAN BEAN SALAD Replace the pasta with 8 ounces fresh string beans, cut into 1½-inch pieces and boiled or steamed until crisp-tender. Replace the spinach and zucchini with 1 can (15 ounces) kidney beans, drained and rinsed. Increase the chickpeas to 1½ cups, or use 1 can (15 ounces) chickpeas, drained and rinsed.

Save for Later

Stored in an airtight container, the pasta salad will keep for 3 days in the refrigerator.

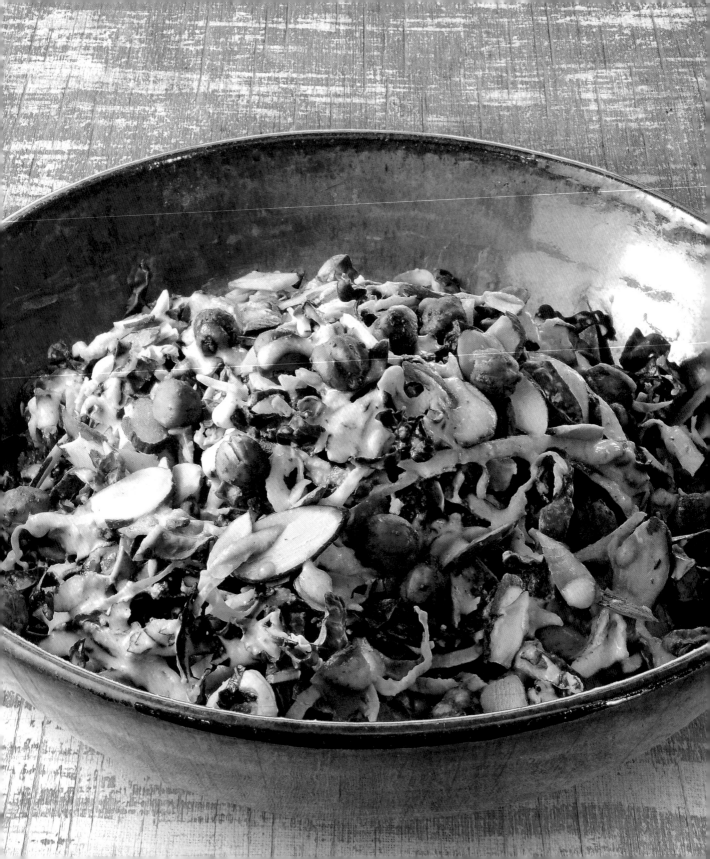

tuscan kale and brussels sprouts caesar salad WITH LEMON-TAHINI DRESSING

Makes 4 servings

Brussels sprouts, kale, and other cruciferous vegetables have high levels of sulfur-containing glucosinolates, which explains their somewhat bitter taste and pungent aroma. But don't let that stop you from enjoying them, as higher intakes have been shown to protect the carotid artery wall. Their crisp and crunchy texture makes them a great addition to any salad, like this Caesar salad that's dressed with a lemony tahini dressing and topped with roasted chickpeas.

LEMON-TAHINI DRESSING (makes 1¼ cups)

½ cup **water**

⅓ cup **tahini**

Juice of 1 **lemon** (¼ cup)

2 tablespoons **hemp seeds**

1 tablespoon reduced-sodium **tamari** or **coconut aminos**

1 large clove **garlic**

SALAD

4 cups stemmed and thinly sliced **Tuscan or curly kale**, lightly packed

1½ cups shredded **green or purple Brussels sprouts**, lightly packed

1 cup thinly sliced **radicchio** or **red cabbage**, lightly packed

1 **carrot**

1 tablespoon **nutritional yeast flakes** or **Almond-Hemp Parmesan** (page 50)

½ cup **Oil-Free Roasted Chickpeas** (page 52)

⅓ cup toasted **sliced almonds,** or 1½ tablespoons **hemp seeds**

1   To make the dressing, put all the ingredients in a blender and process until smooth. Scrape down the blender jar with a silicone spatula and process for 15 seconds longer.

2   To make the salad, put the kale, Brussels sprouts, and radicchio in a large bowl.

3   Use a vegetable peeler to shave long, thin strips down the entire length of the carrot, then coarsely chop the strips into 2-inch long pieces. Add the carrots to the kale mixture and gently toss to combine.

4   Sprinkle the nutritional yeast over the top of the kale mixture. Drizzle ⅔ cup of the dressing over the salad and gently toss until evenly distributed. Scatter the roasted chickpeas and toasted almonds over the top. Drizzle additional dressing over individual servings as desired. Serve immediately.

Save for Later   Stored in separate airtight containers, the dressing will keep for 5 days in the refrigerator and the undressed salad will keep for 3 days in the refrigerator.

TIP   Use a food processor fitted with a thin slicing disc to quickly shred the Brussels sprouts. For easier preparation, use packaged shredded Brussels sprouts, which can be found in the produce section of many grocery stores.

strawberry, avocado, and spinach salad WITH BALSAMIC VINEGAR REDUCTION

Makes 4 servings

When fresh strawberries hit the market, it's the ideal time to make this light and refreshing spinach salad. It's made with juicy strawberries, sweet figs, creamy avocado, crunchy almonds, and a tangy balsamic vinegar reduction—all very simple ingredients, but each one adds a welcome complexity of flavor and texture. For a peppery kick, prepare the salad using half arugula and half spinach.

1 cup **balsamic vinegar**

6 cups **baby spinach**, or 3 cups **baby spinach** and 3 cups **arugula**, lightly packed

2 cups **strawberries**, cut in half and thinly sliced

1 **avocado**, diced

½ small **red onion**, thinly sliced into half-moons

⅓ cup coarsely chopped **dried figs**

⅓ cup **alfalfa sprouts**, lightly packed

⅓ cup raw **sliced almonds** or blanched **slivered almonds**

1   To make the balsamic vinegar reduction, put the vinegar in a small saucepan. Bring to a boil over high heat. Decrease the heat to low and simmer, stirring occasionally, until the vinegar is reduced by one-third to one-half in volume and coats the back of a spoon, about 10 minutes. Remove from the heat. Let cool completely.

2   To make the salad, put the spinach, strawberries, avocado, and onion in a large bowl and toss to combine. Scatter the figs, alfalfa sprouts, and almonds over the top. Drizzle 1 to 2 tablespoons of the balsamic vinegar reduction over individual servings as desired. Serve immediately.

Save for Later   Stored in separate airtight containers, the balsamic vinegar reduction will keep for 2 months in the refrigerator and the salad mixture will keep for 2 days in the refrigerator.

SIDE DISHES

8

beer-braised GREENS

Makes 2 servings

Eating dark leafy greens, such as kale, spinach, and collard greens, on a daily basis can lower the risk of heart disease. That's because they're high in dietary nitrates and vitamin K, both of which have been shown to reduce blood pressure, improve arterial function, and promote blood clotting. Any type of dark leafy green can be used to make this dish, which entails slowly braising the greens in a spicy, beer-based broth.

½ cup diced **yellow onion**

½ cup coarsely chopped **cremini or button mushrooms**

3 large cloves **garlic,** minced

1 bottle (12 ounces) **beer**

1 tablespoon **nutritional yeast flakes**

1½ teaspoons **molasses or brown sugar**

½ teaspoon **smoked paprika** or **chili powder**

1 bunch (1 pound) **leafy greens** (such as collard greens, kale, mustard greens, or turnip greens), **stemmed and thinly sliced**

Sea salt

Freshly ground **black pepper**

Hot sauce or crushed **red pepper flakes** (optional)

1   Put the onion, mushrooms, garlic, and 2 tablespoons of the beer in a large soup pot. Cover and cook over medium-high heat, stirring occasionally, for 5 minutes.

2   Add the remaining beer, nutritional yeast, molasses, and paprika and stir to combine. Bring to a boil over high heat.

3   Add the leafy greens. Cover, decrease the heat to low, and simmer, stirring occasionally, until the greens reach the desired tenderness, 30 to 45 minutes. Season with salt, pepper, and optional hot sauce to taste. Serve hot.

Variation

BEER-BRAISED GREENS WITH BLACK-EYED PEAS When adding the greens, add ¾ cup water and ½ cup dried black-eyed peas, sorted and rinsed. Cook until the black-eyed peas and greens are tender.

Save for Later

Stored in an airtight container, the greens will keep for 5 days in the refrigerator.

FRIJOLES borrachos

Frijoles borrachos literally means "drunken beans" in Spanish. This traditional Mexican dish is made by slow-simmering beans in spices and beer, which adds deep, rich flavor. Recent studies have shown that the barley malt, hops, and yeast used to make beer infuse it with plant sterols, which can help reduce LDL cholesterol. Pile these saucy beans on top of cooked rice or other whole grains or scoop them up with tortilla chips.

1 cup **dried pinto beans,** sorted and rinsed

1 can (14 ounces) **fire-roasted or regular diced tomatoes**

1 bottle (12 ounces) **beer**

1½ cups **water**

¾ cup diced **yellow onion**

¾ cup diced **green bell pepper**

1 **serrano or jalapeño chile,** seeded and finely diced

3 large cloves **garlic,** minced

1 tablespoon **brown sugar** or **coconut sugar**

1 teaspoon **dried oregano**

1 teaspoon **chili powder**

1 teaspoon **ground cumin**

⅓ cup chopped **fresh cilantro,** lightly packed

1 tablespoon **lime juice**

1 tablespoon **nutritional yeast flakes**

Sea salt

Freshly ground **black pepper**

1 Put the beans in a large saucepan or soup pot and cover with warm water. Let soak for 8 to 12 hours. Drain in a colander, rinse the saucepan, and return the beans to the saucepan.

2 Add the tomatoes, beer, water, onion, bell pepper, chile, garlic, brown sugar, oregano, chili powder, and cumin and stir to combine. Bring to a boil over high heat. Cover, decrease the heat to low, and simmer until the beans are soft and most of the liquid has been absorbed, about 1 hour.

3 Using the back of a spoon, mash some of the beans against the side of the saucepan to break them up a bit. Continue to cook until the mixture is slightly thickened, 3 to 5 minutes. Remove from the heat. Add the cilantro, lime juice, and nutritional yeast and stir to combine. Season with salt and pepper to taste. Serve hot.

Save for Later

Stored in an airtight container, the beans will keep for 5 days in the refrigerator or 2 months in the freezer.

sweet potatoes LOADED
WITH BLACK BEAN GUACAMOLE

Makes 2 servings

Guacamole and beans often share the same space inside a burrito. But why not go a different route and give your guacamole a protein boost by adding some black beans to it? And if you love sweet potatoes and chunky guacamole, then these baked beauties, overflowing with guacamole goodness, will quickly become your go-to dish.

1 **Hass avocado,** cut in half

Juice of ½ **lime** (1 tablespoon)

1½ teaspoons **nutritional yeast flakes**

2 large cloves **garlic,** minced

½ teaspoon **chili powder**

⅓ cup cooked **black beans,** drained and rinsed

¼ cup finely diced **red or yellow bell pepper**

2 tablespoons chopped **fresh cilantro,** lightly packed

1 **green onion,** thinly sliced

½ **serrano** or **jalapeño chile,** seeded and finely diced

Sea salt

Freshly ground **black pepper**

2 large **sweet potatoes**

1   To make the guacamole, use a spoon to scoop the avocado out of its skin and put it directly into a medium bowl. Add the lime juice, nutritional yeast, garlic, and chili powder and mash with a fork or potato masher to the desired consistency. Add the beans, bell pepper, cilantro, green onion, and chile and stir to combine. Season with salt and pepper to taste. Cover and store in the refrigerator until ready to serve.

2 To cook the sweet potatoes, preheat the oven to 400 degrees F. Using a fork, pierce each potato in several places on all sides and put them on a baking sheet. Bake for 30 to 40 minutes (turn them over after 20 minutes), until the sweet potatoes are soft and can be easily squeezed. Alternatively, to cook the pierced sweet potatoes in the microwave, put them in a glass or ceramic baking pan and microwave for 10 to 15 minutes, until the sweet potatoes are soft.

3 Using a sharp knife, cut a slit down the length of each sweet potato. Gently squeeze the sides toward the middle to open the sweet potatoes, then put them on a large platter or on individual plates. Alternatively, cut each potato in half lengthwise and put them cut-side up on a platter or plate.

4 Top each sweet potato with half of the guacamole. Serve hot.

Variation

OVERLOADED BAKED SWEET POTATOES Spoon ⅓ cup Creamy Cauliflower Cheese Sauce (page 56) or Cauliflower Queso Dip (see page 56) over the top of each sweet potato before topping with the guacamole.

Variation

Replace the sweet potatoes with large russet potatoes, or forego the potatoes altogether and just dig into the guacamole with tortilla chips.

Save for Later

Stored in separate airtight containers, the guacamole and baked sweet potatoes will keep for 3 days in the refrigerator.

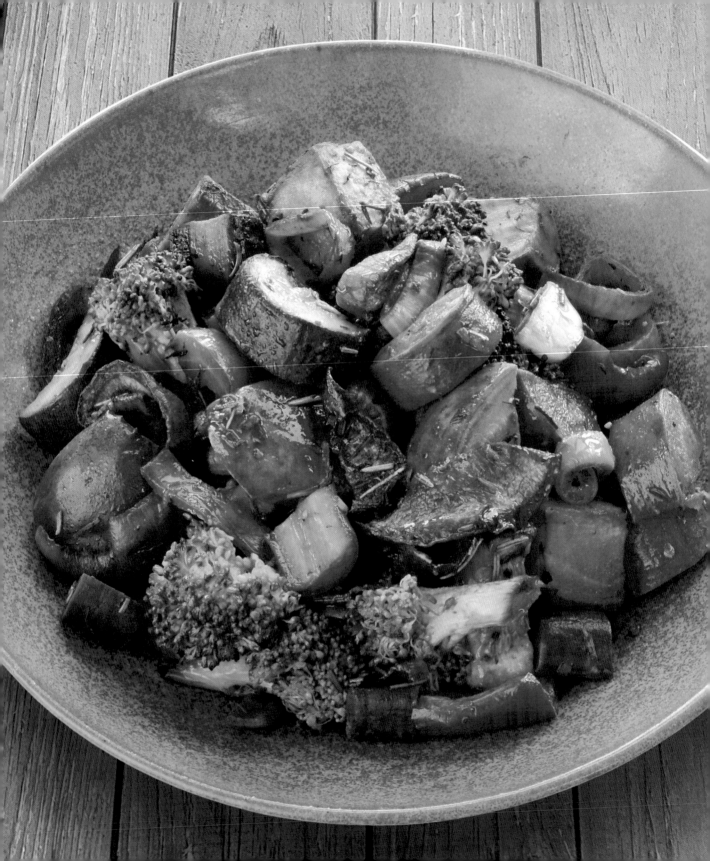

RAINBOW roasted vegetables

Makes 4 servings

The American Heart Association recommends eating eight or more servings of fruits and vegetables every day. As a result, "eat the rainbow" has become a popular healthy-eating slogan to remind people to include a colorful assortment of fruits and veggies in their daily diets. This recipe features vegetables in every hue of the rainbow, which makes it quite an eye-catching side dish.

1½ cups **broccoli,** cut into small florets, or 1 bunch (8 ounces) **broccolini,** cut into 1-inch pieces

3 **carrots** (preferably multicolored), cut in half lengthwise and sliced ½ inch thick

1 large **golden beet** or **parsnip,** peeled and cut into 1-inch cubes

1 large **red onion,** cut into ¼-inch-thick half-moons

1 **orange or yellow bell pepper,** cut into 1 x ½-inch pieces

1 **red bell pepper,** cut into 1 x ½-inch pieces

1 **zucchini,** cut in half lengthwise and sliced into ½-inch-thick half-moons

1½ tablespoons **balsamic vinegar**

1½ tablespoons reduced-sodium **tamari** or **coconut aminos**

1½ tablespoons **nutritional yeast flakes**

1 teaspoon **dried basil**

1 teaspoon **dried oregano**

1 teaspoon **dried thyme** or **rosemary**

½ teaspoon crushed **red pepper flakes** (optional)

Sea salt

Freshly ground **black pepper**

1 Preheat the oven to 400 degrees F. Line a baking sheet with parchment paper or a silicone baking mat.

2   Put the broccoli, carrots, beet, onion, orange bell pepper, red bell pepper, zucchini, vinegar, tamari, nutritional yeast, basil, oregano, thyme, and optional red pepper flakes in a large bowl and stir until the vegetables are evenly coated.

3   Transfer to the lined baking sheet and spread into a single layer. Season with salt and pepper to taste. Bake for 25 to 35 minutes, until the vegetables are tender and lightly browned around the edges. Serve hot.

Variation   Replace the suggested vegetables with other rainbow-colored vegetables, such as red or chioggia beets, Brussels sprouts, cauliflower, potatoes, sweet potatoes, winter squash, or yellow summer squash. To ensure even cooking, cut the vegetables into bite-sized pieces.

Save for Later   Stored in an airtight container, the roasted vegetables will keep for 3 days in the refrigerator.

BUTTERY mashed potatoes

Makes 4 servings

Although there's no butter in these mashed potatoes, there are butter beans, which are plump, light-colored lima beans. Cooked butter beans have a very soft skin and creamy interior, which makes them the ideal butter-free partner for these tasty taters. Serve them plain or topped with Quick Cashew Gravy (page 57) or Creamy Cauliflower Cheese Sauce (page 56).

2 pounds **Yukon gold potatoes,** peeled and cut into 2-inch cubes

1 can (15 ounces) **butter beans,** drained and rinsed

3 large cloves **garlic,** thinly sliced

1 cup plain **soy milk, oat milk,** or other **nondairy milk**

3 tablespoons **nutritional yeast flakes** or **Almond-Hemp Parmesan** (page 50)

Sea salt

Freshly ground **black pepper** or **white pepper**

1 Put the potatoes in a large saucepan or soup pot and cover with water. Cook over medium-high heat for 15 minutes.

2 Add the beans and garlic and cook, stirring occasionally, until the potatoes are soft, 5 to 10 minutes.

3 Drain in a colander. Rinse the saucepan and return the potato mixture to the saucepan.

4 Add the milk and nutritional yeast. Mash the potatoes with a potato masher until they are as smooth as you like. Season with salt and pepper to taste. Serve hot.

Save for Later | Stored in an airtight container, the mashed potatoes will keep for 3 days in the refrigerator.

golden barley WITH VEGETABLES

Makes 4 servings

Barley has a slightly nutty flavor and chewy texture that makes it an outstanding choice for adding bulk to soups, stews, salads, or side dishes. Although it can be steamed much like rice, due to barley's high starch content, the individual grains tend to clump together. To avoid that, cook barley like pasta by boiling it in plenty of water and then draining it in a strainer once it's tender.

6 cups **water**

1 cup **hulled or pearl barley**, rinsed

1 small **leek**, cut in half lengthwise and thinly sliced, or ¾ cup diced **yellow onion**

1 **carrot,** finely diced

1 stalk **celery,** finely diced

¼ cup low-sodium **vegetable broth** or additional **water**

2 large cloves **garlic,** minced

2 teaspoons **dried thyme**

1½ teaspoons **dried dill weed** or **basil**

¾ cup frozen **peas** or **edamame,** thawed

⅓ cup **white wine** (such as Chardonnay or Riesling)

2 tablespoons **nutritional yeast flakes** or **Almond-Hemp Parmesan** (page 50)

½ teaspoon **ground turmeric** or **curry powder**

⅓ cup chopped **fresh parsley,** lightly packed

Sea salt

Freshly ground **black pepper**

1. To cook the barley, put the water in a large saucepan. Bring to a boil over medium-high heat. Add the barley and cook, stirring occasionally, until the barley is tender, 30 to 45 minutes depending on the variety. Drain the barley in a fine-mesh strainer, rinse with cold water, and drain again.

2. While the barley is cooking, make the vegetable mixture. Put the leek, carrot, celery, broth, garlic, thyme, and dill weed in a large nonstick skillet and cook over medium-high heat, stirring occasionally, until the vegetables are soft, 8 to 10 minutes. Add the peas and cook, stirring occasionally, for 2 minutes.

3. Add the cooked barley and wine, nutritional yeast, and turmeric and cook, stirring constantly, until the wine has been absorbed and the barley turns yellow, 1 to 2 minutes. Add the parsley and stir until evenly distributed. Season with salt and pepper to taste. Serve hot.

Save for Later

Stored in an airtight container, the barley and vegetables will keep for 3 days in the refrigerator.

lentil and rice PILAF

Makes 4 servings

Eating folate-rich foods, such as lentils, every day can help reduce the risk of cardiovascular disease. Lentils and rice are a popular pairing in dishes eaten around the world. In this pilaf they are combined with seasonings used in Mediterranean and Middle Eastern cuisines, along with iron-rich greens and aromatic vegetables. This savory side can also be used as a filling for stuffed and baked bell peppers or winter squash.

4 cups **water,** or 2 cups water and 2 cups low-sodium **vegetable broth**

1 cup **dried brown lentils,** sorted and rinsed

1 cup **long-grain brown rice,** or 1 cup **long-grain and mixed-rice blend**

1 cup diced **carrot**

1 cup diced **yellow onion**

1 stalk **celery,** cut in half lengthwise and thinly sliced

3 large cloves **garlic,** minced

2 teaspoons **dried basil**

1½ teaspoons **dried thyme** or **rosemary**

1 teaspoon **ground cumin**

1 teaspoon **ground coriander**

2 cups coarsely chopped **spinach,** lightly packed

⅓ cup chopped **fresh parsley** or **cilantro,** lightly packed

1½ tablespoons reduced-sodium **tamari** or **coconut aminos**

Sea salt

Freshly ground **black pepper**

1   Put the water, lentils, rice, carrot, onion, celery, garlic, basil, thyme, cumin, and coriander in a large saucepan and stir to combine. Bring to a boil over high heat. Cover, decrease the heat to low, and simmer until the lentils and rice are tender and all of the water is absorbed, 35 to 45 minutes. Remove from the heat.

2   Put the spinach on top of the lentil mixture, cover, and let sit for 5 minutes to allow the spinach to wilt slightly. Add the parsley and tamari and stir until evenly distributed. Season with salt and pepper to taste. Serve hot.

Variation

CELEBRATION LENTIL AND RICE PILAF Replace the carrot with 1½ cups peeled and diced sweet potatoes. When adding the spinach, also add ⅓ cup dried cranberries and ⅓ cup coarsely chopped nuts (such as almonds, hazelnuts, pecans, or walnuts).

Save for Later

Stored in an airtight container, the rice pilaf will keep for 3 days in the refrigerator.

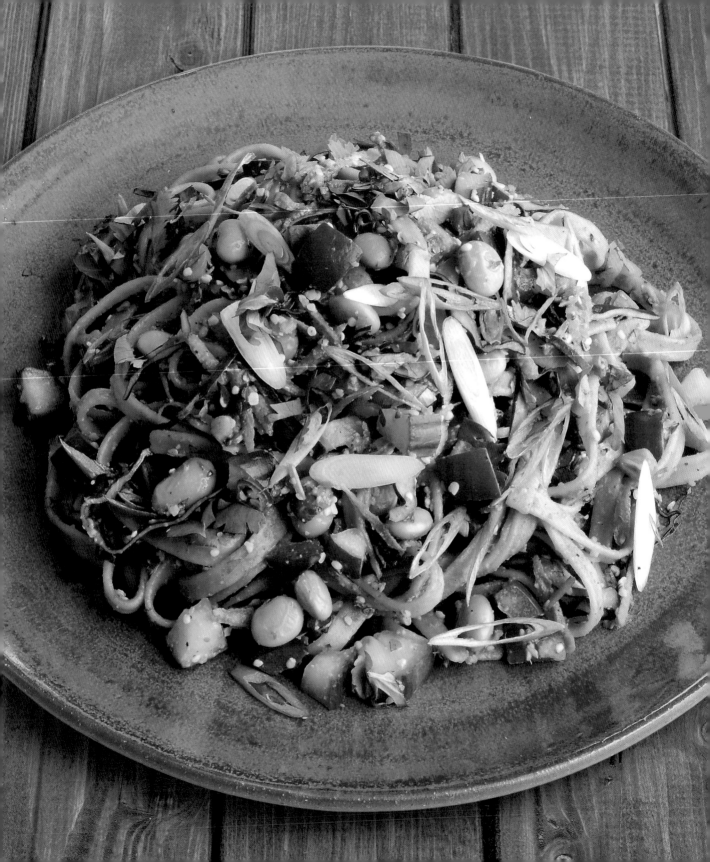

edamame and vegetable
SZECHUAN NOODLES

Makes 4 servings

The vibrant green color of the plump edamame (immature soy beans) complements the crisp raw vegetables and chewy noodles in this salad, which are coated with a spicy nut butter sauce. This makes a tasty side dish, or serve it as a main dish on top of shredded leafy greens, accompanied by steamed broccoli.

¼ cup **peanut butter, almond butter,** or **tahini**

3 tablespoons reduced-sodium **tamari** or **coconut aminos**

2 tablespoons **coconut sugar** or **brown sugar**

Juice of 1 **lime** (2 tablespoons)

1 tablespoon minced **garlic**

1 tablespoon peeled and grated **fresh ginger**

½ teaspoon crushed **red pepper flakes** (optional)

¼ teaspoon freshly ground **black pepper**

8 ounces **brown rice** or **whole-grain thin noodles** (such as spaghetti, linguine, or soba)

1 cup frozen shelled **edamame,** thawed

1 cup shredded **red cabbage**

¾ cup shredded **carrot**

½ cup diced **red or orange bell pepper**

¼ cup seeded and finely diced **cucumber**

¼ cup thinly sliced **green onions**

¼ cup chopped **fresh cilantro** or **parsley,** lightly packed

1½ tablespoons **hemp seeds** or **sesame seeds**

1   To make the sauce, put the peanut butter, tamari, sugar, lime juice, garlic, ginger, optional red pepper flakes, and pepper in a small bowl and stir to combine.

2 Cook the noodles in boiling water according to the package directions. Drain in a colander, rinse with cold water, and drain again. Transfer to a large bowl.

3 Add the sauce and gently toss to evenly coat the noodles. Add the edamame, cabbage, carrot, bell pepper, cucumber, green onions, cilantro, and hemp seeds and gently toss until evenly distributed. Serve cold or at room temperature.

Variation

EDAMAME AND VEGETABLE SZECHUAN ZOODLES Replace the cooked noodles with 2 large zucchini that have been cut into noodle shapes with a spiralizer or vegetable peeler. Do not cook the zucchini noodles.

Save for Later

Stored in an airtight container, the Szechuan noodles will keep for 3 days in the refrigerator.

MAIN DISHES

9

HEMP falafel burgers

Hemp seeds and oat bran work beautifully as binders and also add an extra boost of fiber and omega-3s to these protein-packed falafel patties, which are oven-baked instead of deep-fried. Serve them on buns with your favorite toppings and condiments, or make classic falafel sandwiches by tucking them into pita pockets with sliced tomatoes and cucumbers and drizzling the tops with Lemon-Tahini Dressing (page 75).

½ small **yellow onion,** cut into four pieces

3 large cloves **garlic**

¼ cup **fresh parsley** leaves, lightly packed

¼ cup **fresh mint** or **cilantro leaves,** lightly packed

2 tablespoons **lemon juice**

1 tablespoon **tahini**

1 teaspoon **ground cumin**

1 teaspoon **ground coriander**

½ teaspoon **sweet or smoked paprika**

½ teaspoon **sea salt**

¼ teaspoon freshly ground **black pepper**

1 can (15-ounces) **chickpeas,** drained and rinsed

¼ cup **hemp seeds**

¼ cup **oat bran**

1 Put the onion, garlic, parsley, and mint in a food processor and process until finely chopped. Scrape down the work bowl with a silicone spatula. Add the lemon juice, tahini, cumin, coriander, paprika, salt, and pepper and process for 15 seconds. Add the chickpeas and pulse until the chickpeas are coarsely chopped.

2 Transfer to a medium bowl. Add the hemp seeds and oat bran and work them in with your hands until evenly distributed and the mixture holds together when squeezed.

3 Shape into four patties and put them on a large plate. Flatten each patty into a 4-inch circle. Refrigerate for 30 minutes to let the patties firm up slightly.

4 Preheat the oven to 400 degrees F. Line a baking sheet with parchment paper or a silicone baking mat.

5 Transfer the patties to the lined baking sheet and bake for 20 minutes. Remove from the oven and flip the patties over with a metal spatula. Bake for 10 to 15 minutes longer, or until golden brown on both sides. Serve immediately.

Save for Later   Stored in an airtight container, the falafel burgers will keep for 3 days in the refrigerator.

bean and rice BURRITOS

Burritos are incredibly versatile, as they can be served for breakfast, lunch, or dinner, or even as a late-night snack. These hearty burritos are made with layers of seasoned beans, cilantro, lime-flavored rice, avocado, queso dip, salsa, and shredded lettuce. Serve them right away, wrap them up for an on-the-go meal, or elevate them to the next level by putting them on a plate and smothering them with additional queso dip and salsa.

½ cup diced **red or yellow onion**

2 large cloves **garlic,** minced

2 tablespoons **water**

1 can (15 ounces) **beans** (black, kidney, pinto, or red), drained and rinsed

1 tablespoon **chili powder**

1 teaspoon **ground cumin**

1 teaspoon **hot sauce**

1 teaspoon **nutritional yeast flakes**

2 cups cooked **brown or white rice** or other **whole grains** (such as millet or quinoa)

⅓ cup chopped **fresh cilantro** or **parsley,** lightly packed

Juice and zest of 1 **lime** (2 teaspoons zest and 2 tablespoons juice)

Sea salt

Freshly ground **black pepper**

4 (8-inch or larger) **whole-grain or flour tortillas**

1 **avocado,** sliced

½ cup **Cauliflower Queso Dip** (see page 56)

1 cup **Mango-Pineapple Salsa** (page 48), or ½ cup **salsa**

4 large **lettuce leaves** (such as looseleaf or romaine), shredded

1 Put the onion, garlic, and water in a large nonstick skillet and cook over medium-high heat, stirring occasionally, until the onion is soft, about 5 minutes. Add the beans, chili powder, cumin, hot sauce, and nutritional yeast and cook, stirring occasionally, until the beans are heated through, 3 to 5 minutes. Remove from the heat.

2 Put the rice in a small bowl. Add the cilantro and lime zest and juice and stir until evenly distributed. Season with salt and pepper to taste.

3   For easier rolling, warm each tortilla in a large nonstick skillet over medium heat for 1 minute per side. Alternatively, warm the tortillas in the microwave for 20 to 30 seconds.

4   To assemble each burrito, put a tortilla on a large plate. Spoon ⅓ cup of the bean mixture and ½ cup of the rice mixture horizontally in the center of the tortilla. Top with one-quarter of the sliced avocado, 2 tablespoons Cauliflower Queso Dip, ¼ cup Mango-Pineapple Salsa, and one-quarter of the shredded lettuce.

5   To roll the burrito, fold the bottom half of the tortilla over the filling, fold in each side toward the center over the filling, and roll up from the bottom edge to enclose the filling.

Save for Later

Stored seam-side down in an airtight container or wrapped in plastic wrap or aluminum foil, the burritos will keep for 2 days in the refrigerator.

oat bran–breaded tofu or tempeh CUTLETS

The coarse texture of oat bran and almond flour makes them excellent substitutes for bread crumbs. For this healthier version of vegan fried chicken, they're combined with hemp seeds, nutritional yeast, and spices to make a seasoned breading mixture for marinated tofu or tempeh. Serve these cutlets plain or with gravy, or as a high-protein filling for sandwiches and wraps. When cut into smaller pieces, they make a tasty addition to salads or soups.

1 pound extra-firm **tofu,** pressed (see page 69), **or 2 packages** (8 ounces) **tempeh**

½ cup plain **soy milk** or other **nondairy milk**

1½ tablespoons reduced-sodium **tamari**

1 tablespoon **balsamic vinegar**

Several drops **hot sauce**

½ cup **oat bran**

¼ cup **almond flour**

2 tablespoons **hemp seeds**

2 tablespoons **nutritional yeast flakes**

1 teaspoon **garlic granules**

1 teaspoon **onion powder**

1 teaspoon **dried basil**

1 teaspoon **dried thyme**

1 teaspoon **sweet or smoked paprika**

½ teaspoon **sea salt**

½ teaspoon freshly ground **black pepper**

1 If using tofu, cut it lengthwise into eight slices. If using tempeh, cut each package of tempeh into four slices. Arrange the slices in a single layer in an 11 x 7-inch baking pan. Using a fork, pierce each slice several times along its length. Flip each slice over and pierce the other side.

2   To make the marinade, put the milk, tamari, vinegar, and hot sauce in a small bowl and stir to combine. Pour over the tofu or tempeh and flip over each slice to evenly coat all sides. Put the baking pan in the refrigerator and let the slices marinate for at least 1 hour.

3   To make the breading, put the oat bran, almond flour, hemp seeds, nutritional yeast, garlic granules, onion powder, basil, thyme, paprika, salt, and pepper on a large plate and toss with your fingers to combine.

4   Preheat the oven to 400 degrees F. Line a baking sheet with parchment paper or a silicone baking mat.

5   To coat the tofu or tempeh, work with one slice at a time. Put each slice into the breading mixture, pressing down slightly and flipping the slice over as needed to evenly coat all sides. Transfer to the lined baking sheet.

6   Bake for 20 minutes. Remove from the oven and flip the cutlets over. Bake for 15 to 20 minutes longer, until lightly browned on both sides. Serve hot.

Save for Later   Stored in an airtight container, the cutlets will keep for 3 days in the refrigerator.

sheet-pan SUPPER

A sheet-pan supper is ideal for hectic days, as it can be quickly assembled and then tossed in the oven. It's also a great way to use up veggies, beans, or other ingredients in your pantry or fridge. Serve it with cooked whole grains, rice, or pasta, or on a bed of leafy greens. For even more richness and flavor, drizzle each serving with a little Lemon-Tahini Dressing or Yogurt Ranch Dressing.

1 can (15 ounces) **chickpeas,** drained and rinsed

Juice of 1 **lime** (2 tablespoons)

2 tablespoons reduced-sodium **tamari**

2 tablespoons **water**

1 teaspoon **garlic granules**

1 teaspoon **onion powder**

1 teaspoon **dried basil**

1 teaspoon **dried oregano**

1 teaspoon **curry powder** or **chili powder**

1 teaspoon **sweet or smoked paprika**

1 small head **white, orange, or purple cauliflower** or **Romanesco,** cut into small florets

1 **delicata squash,** seeded and cut into 1-inch cubes, or 1 large **sweet potato,** cut into 1-inch cubes

1½ cups cubed **red-skinned potatoes** or quartered **small potatoes**

1 **orange, red, or yellow bell pepper,** cut into 1 x ½-inch pieces

8 ounces extra-firm **tofu,** pressed (see page 69) and cut into 1 x ½-inch strips, or 1 package (8 ounces) **tempeh** cut into 1-inch cubes

2 tablespoons **nutritional yeast flakes** or **Almond-Hemp Parmesan** (page 50)

Sea salt

Freshly ground **black pepper**

¾ cup to 1 cup **Lemon-Tahini Dressing** (page 75; optional) or **Yogurt Ranch Dressing** (page 115; optional)

1 Transfer ½ cup of the chickpeas to an airtight container and refrigerate for use in another recipe. Let the remaining chickpeas air-dry for 15 minutes.

2 Preheat the oven to 400 degrees F. Line a baking sheet with parchment paper or a silicone baking mat.

3   To make the marinade, put the lime juice, tamari, water, garlic granules, onion powder, basil, oregano, curry powder, and paprika in a small bowl and whisk to combine.

4   Put the cauliflower, squash, potatoes, and bell pepper in a large bowl. Add the tofu and chickpeas and stir to combine. Pour the marinade over the top and stir until the vegetables and tofu are evenly coated.

5   Transfer to the lined baking sheet and spread into a single layer. Sprinkle the nutritional yeast evenly over the top and season with salt and pepper.

6   Bake for 40 to 45 minutes, until the vegetables are tender and lightly browned around the edges. Drizzle each serving with 3 to 4 tablespoons of the optional dressing. Serve hot.

Variation Replace the suggested vegetables with other vegetables, such as beets, broccoli or broccolini, Brussels sprouts, yellow summer squash, or zucchini. To ensure even cooking, cut the vegetables into bite-sized pieces.

Save for Later Stored in an airtight container, the vegetable mixture will keep for 3 days in the refrigerator.

roasted chestnut and mushroom **BOURGUIGNON**

The resveratrol in red wine can help reduce inflammation in the body, prevent damage to blood vessels, and lower LDL cholesterol. Adding a bit of wine to a recipe can make it taste great too! For this meatless version of the classic French stew, aromatic vegetables, earthy mushrooms, and roasted chestnuts are simmered in red wine and vegetable broth. Serve it with whole-grain bread or a side of Buttery Mashed Potatoes (page 87), or spoon it over pasta, rice, or whole grains.

12 ounces **cremini or button mushrooms,** cut into quarters

1 **yellow onion,** diced

2 **carrots,** cut in half lengthwise and sliced ½ inch thick

¼ cup **water**

4 large cloves **garlic,** minced

¼ cup **oat flour** (see page 45) or **barley flour**

2 cups **red wine** (such as Burgundy or Pinot Noir)

2 cups low-sodium **vegetable broth** or **mushroom broth**

1 package (3.5 ounces) peeled and roasted **chestnuts,** thinly sliced

1 tablespoon **tomato paste** or **ketchup**

1 **bay leaf**

1½ teaspoons **dried basil**

1½ teaspoons **dried thyme** or **rosemary**

¼ cup chopped **fresh parsley,** lightly packed

2 tablespoons **nutritional yeast flakes**

1 tablespoon **balsamic vinegar** or **Balsamic Vinegar Reduction** (see page 77)

Sea salt

Freshly ground **black pepper**

1. Put the mushrooms, onion, carrots, water, and garlic in a large soup pot. Cover and cook over medium-high heat, stirring occasionally, until the vegetables are soft, 8 to 10 minutes.

2. Sprinkle the flour over the mushroom mixture and cook, stirring occasionally, for 1 minute.

3. Add the wine, broth, chestnuts, tomato paste, bay leaf, basil, and thyme and stir to combine. Bring to a boil over high heat. Cover, decrease the heat to low, and simmer, stirring occasionally, until the mushrooms are tender and the stew has thickened, 25 to 30 minutes.

4. Remove and discard the bay leaf. Remove from the heat. Add the parsley, nutritional yeast, and vinegar and stir until evenly distributed. Season with salt and pepper to taste. Serve hot.

Save for Later

Stored in an airtight container, the bourguignon will keep for 5 days in the refrigerator or 2 months in the freezer.

ratatouille

Nightshade vegetables, such as eggplant, peppers, potatoes, and tomatoes, were once thought to increase arthritis symptoms, but recent research has shown otherwise. Their consumption is now encouraged for anyone following an anti-inflammatory diet plan. One of the most famous nightshade-based dishes is ratatouille, a classic French vegetable stew. Serve it with whole-grain bread, or, for an even heartier meal, ladle it over cooked pasta or polenta.

1 **eggplant** (1 pound), cut into 2-inch cubes

1 **orange or yellow bell pepper,** cut into 1 x ½-inch pieces

1 **red bell pepper,** cut into 1 x ½-inch pieces

1 **yellow onion,** diced

1 **zucchini** or **yellow summer squash,** cut in half lengthwise and sliced ½ inch thick

1½ tablespoons **minced garlic**

1¾ cups **tomato broth** or **water**

2 large **tomatoes,** diced, or 1 can (14 ounces) **diced tomatoes** (do not drain)

1 tablespoon **balsamic or red wine vinegar**

1 teaspoon **dried basil**

1 teaspoon **dried oregano** or **marjoram**

¼ cup chopped **fresh parsley** or **basil,** lightly packed

2 tablespoons **nutritional yeast flakes** or **Almond-Hemp Parmesan** (page 50)

Sea salt

Freshly ground **black pepper**

1 Put the eggplant, orange bell pepper, red bell pepper, onion, zucchini, and garlic in a large soup pot. Add ¼ cup of the broth and cook over medium-high heat, stirring occasionally, for 7 minutes.

2 Add the remaining 1½ cups broth and the tomatoes, vinegar, basil, and oregano and stir to combine. Bring to a boil over high heat. Cover, decrease the heat to low, and simmer, stirring occasionally, until the vegetables are tender, 20 to 25 minutes.

3 Add the parsley and nutritional yeast and stir until evenly distributed. Season with salt and pepper to taste. Serve hot.

Save for Later | Stored in an airtight container, the ratatouille will keep for 5 days in the refrigerator or 2 months in the freezer.

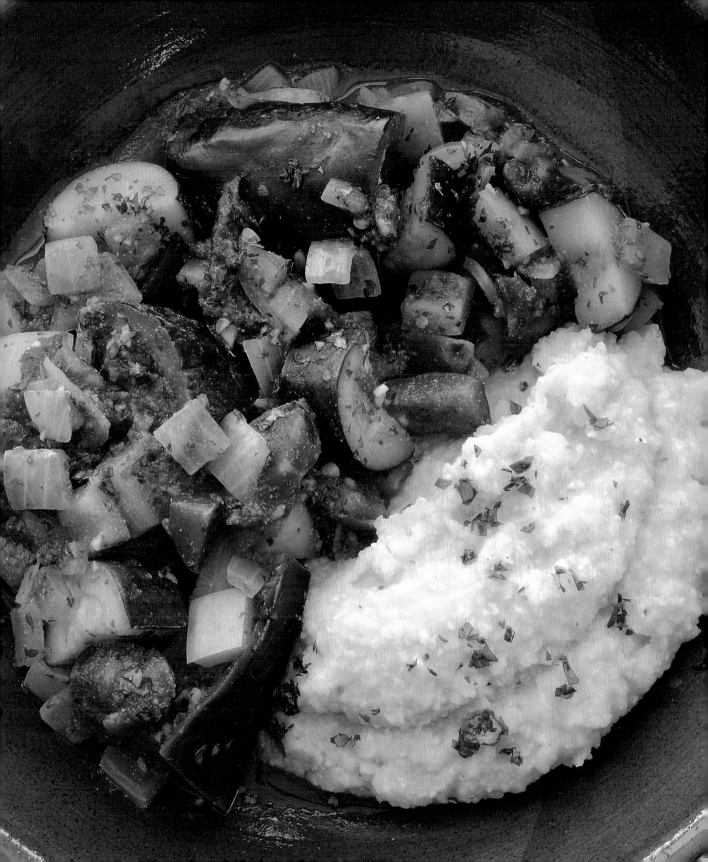

tempeh bolognese
WITH MUSHROOMS AND RED WINE

Makes 6 cups, 6 servings

Protein-rich soy products, such as tofu and soy milk, can help lower LDL cholesterol. But don't overlook tempeh, as it also supplies beneficial probiotics and prebiotics and is easier to digest. In this meatless version of classic Italian Bolognese, crumbled bits of tempeh are combined with chewy mushrooms to create a thick and hearty sauce. Serve it over polenta or pasta with a sprinkling of nutritional yeast flakes or Almond-Hemp Parmesan.

1 package (8 ounces) **tempeh**

1 **yellow onion,** diced

1½ cups coarsely chopped **cremini or white button mushrooms**

4 large cloves **garlic,** minced

¾ cup **water**

1 tablespoon reduced-sodium **tamari**

1 can (28 ounces) **fire-roasted or regular crushed tomatoes**

1 can (8 ounces) **tomato sauce**

⅓ cup **red wine** (such as Burgundy or Pinot Noir)

1 **bay leaf**

1½ teaspoons **dried basil**

1½ teaspoons **dried oregano**

¼ teaspoon crushed **red pepper flakes**

¼ cup chopped **fresh parsley,** lightly packed

1 tablespoon **nutritional yeast flakes** or **Almond-Hemp Parmesan** (page 50)

Sea salt

Freshly ground **black pepper**

1 Using your fingers, crumble the tempeh into small pieces and set aside.

2 Put the onion, mushrooms, and garlic in a large soup pot. Cover and cook over medium-high heat, stirring occasionally, until the onion is soft, about 5 minutes.

3 Add the tempeh, ¼ cup of the water, and the tamari and bring to a boil over high heat. Cover, decrease the heat to low, and simmer for 5 minutes. Remove the lid and continue to cook, stirring occasionally, until the liquid has evaporated and the tempeh has browned slightly, 1 to 2 minutes.

4 Add the crushed tomatoes, tomato sauce, remaining ½ cup of water, and the wine, bay leaf, basil, oregano, and red pepper flakes and stir to combine. Cover, decrease the heat to low, and simmer, stirring occasionally, for 10 to 15 minutes.

5 Remove and discard the bay leaf. Remove from the heat. Add the parsley and nutritional yeast and stir until evenly distributed. Season with salt and pepper to taste. Serve hot.

Variation

Replace the dried basil with ¼ cup chopped fresh basil, lightly packed.

Save for Later

Stored in an airtight container, the Bolognese will keep for 5 days in the refrigerator or 2 months in the freezer.

lemony pasta WITH
ARTICHOKES, BEANS, AND SPINACH

Makes 4 servings

Citrus fruits are high in vitamin C and heart-healthy soluble fiber. Adding more of them to meals can help lower blood glucose levels, blood pressure levels, and LDL cholesterol. For this light main dish, pasta, artichokes, and spinach are cloaked in a simple sauce made of white wine, lemon zest and juice, and fresh herbs. The final addition of hemp seeds, almond flour, and Almond-Hemp Parmesan gives the dish a rich, buttery taste without adding any butter.

8 ounces **whole-grain or bean-based pasta** (such as linguine, penne, rotini, spaghetti, or ziti)

1 cup thawed frozen or canned (packed in water) **artichoke hearts,** drained and coarsely chopped

½ cup diced **shallots,** or ¾ cup diced **yellow onion**

4 large cloves **garlic,** thinly sliced

2 to 4 tablespoons **water,** as needed

4 cups coarsely chopped **baby spinach,** lightly packed

1 cup cooked or canned **cannellini beans** or **chickpeas,** drained and rinsed

½ cup **white wine** (such as Chardonnay or Riesling)

⅓ cup chopped **fresh basil** or **parsley,** lightly packed

Zest and juice of 1 **lemon** (1½ teaspoons zest and ¼ cup juice)

2 tablespoons **Almond-Hemp Parmesan** (page 50) or **nutritional yeast flakes,** plus more for garnish

2 tablespoons **hemp seeds**

2 tablespoons **almond flour**

Sea salt

Freshly ground **black pepper**

Crushed **red pepper flakes**

1 Cook the pasta in boiling water according to the package directions. Drain in a colander, rinse under cold water, and drain again.

2 While the pasta is boiling, cook the vegetables. Put the artichokes, shallots, garlic, and 2 tablespoons water in a large nonstick skillet and cook over medium heat, stirring occasionally, for 5 minutes. Add an additional 1 to 2 tablespoons water as needed to prevent the vegetables from sticking to the bottom of the skillet.

3 Add the spinach and beans and cook, stirring occasionally, until the spinach has wilted, 1 to 2 minutes.

4 Add the cooked pasta, wine, basil, and lemon zest and juice and cook, stirring occasionally, for 1 minute longer to blend the flavors. Remove from the heat.

5 Add the Parmesan, hemp seeds, and almond flour and gently toss until evenly distributed. Season with salt, pepper, and red pepper flakes to taste. Garnish each serving with additional Parmesan. Serve hot.

Variation

LEMONY PASTA WITH ASPARAGUS, BEANS, AND SPINACH Replace the artichokes with 1½ cups trimmed and diagonally sliced asparagus (1-inch pieces).

Save for Later

Stored in an airtight container, the pasta will keep for 3 days in the refrigerator.

cheesy millet and vegetable
casserole WITH ALMOND CRUMB TOPPING

Makes 6 servings

Whole-grain millet is an excellent source of magnesium, which has been shown to help lower high blood pressure, slow the progression of atherosclerosis, and reduce the risk of heart attack. Millet's mild flavor also makes it a viable alternative to rice and other cooked grains. This comfort-food casserole takes a little advance planning, but it can be assembled ahead of time, so all you have to do is pop it in the oven shortly before serving.

½ cup **millet,** rinsed

1 cup **water**

1 pound **broccoli,** cut into small florets, or 8 ounces **broccoli** and 8 ounces **cauliflower,** cut into small florets

½ cup diced **orange or red bell pepper**

½ cup thinly sliced **green onions**

2 cups **Creamy Cauliflower Cheese Sauce** (page 56)

1½ cups coarsely chopped **baby spinach,** lightly packed

¼ cup chopped **fresh parsley,** lightly packed

Sea salt

Freshly ground **black pepper**

2 tablespoons **almond flour**

1 tablespoon **oat bran**

1 tablespoon **nutritional yeast flakes** or **Almond-Hemp Parmesan** (page 50)

Sweet or smoked paprika

1 Preheat the oven to 375 degrees F. Lightly mist an 11 x 7-inch baking pan with cooking spray.

2 To toast the millet, put it in a medium saucepan and cook over medium heat, stirring occasionally, until the grains begin to "pop" and are lightly browned, 1 to 2 minutes.

3. Add the water and bring to a boil over high heat. Cover, decrease the heat to low, and simmer until the millet is tender and all of the water is absorbed, 20 to 25 minutes.

4. While the millet is cooking, prebake the vegetables. Put the broccoli and bell pepper in the prepared baking pan and spread into a single layer. Bake for 15 to 18 minutes, until the broccoli is tender and slightly browned around the edges. Scatter the green onions over the top and bake for 2 minutes longer, until slightly wilted. Remove from the oven. Using a metal spatula, loosen the vegetables from the bottom and sides of the baking pan and set aside.

5. Fluff the millet with a fork to separate the grains. Add the cheese sauce, spinach, and parsley and stir to combine. Add the millet mixture to the broccoli mixture and stir until evenly combined. Season with salt and pepper to taste. Smooth the top of the casserole with the back of a spoon or a silicone spatula.

6. Put the almond flour, oat bran, and nutritional yeast in a small bowl and stir to combine. Scatter the almond flour mixture evenly over the millet mixture. Sprinkle a little paprika over the top.

7. Bake for 15 to 18 minutes, until the casserole is heated through and the topping is lightly browned. Remove from the oven. Let sit for 5 minutes before serving. Serve hot.

Save for Later   Stored in an airtight container, the casserole will keep for 3 days in the refrigerator.

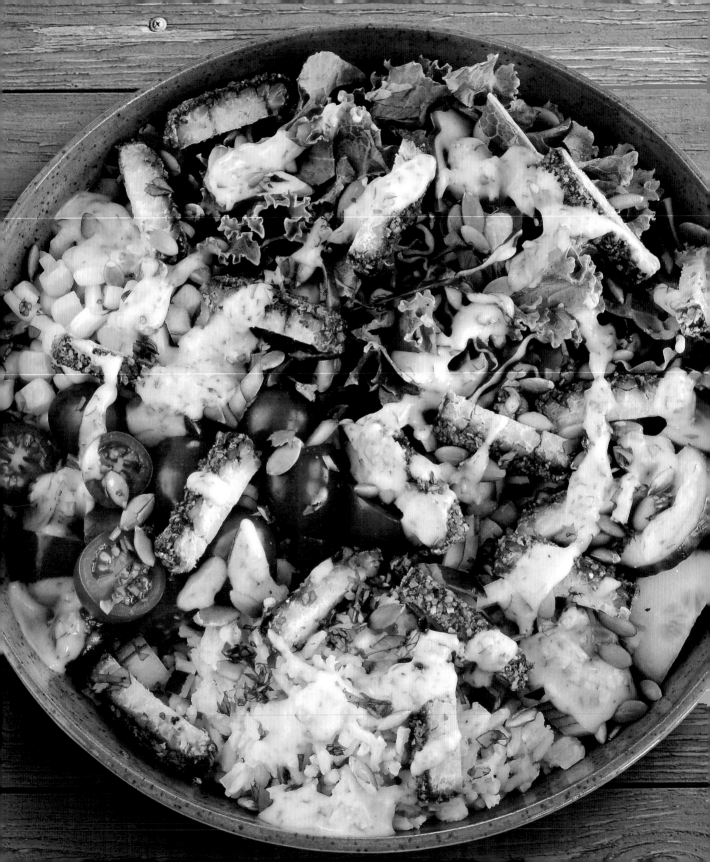

grain and garden buddha bowls
WITH YOGURT RANCH DRESSING

Makes 4 servings

Buddha bowls—the eye-catching main-dish meals that are commonly served in large, wide bowls—are made by artistically arranging or layering a combination of ingredients. To create yours, start with a cooked grain, then add a mix of raw and cooked vegetables, leafy greens, and a plant-based protein (beans, lentils, tempeh, or tofu). Sprinkle with nuts or seeds and drizzle with a flavorful dressing or sauce. Now you have a main-dish masterpiece!

YOGURT RANCH DRESSING (makes 1⅓ cups)

⅔ cup plain **oat yogurt** or other **nondairy yogurt**

½ cup plain **oat milk** or **soy milk**

3 tablespoons **cider vinegar**

2 tablespoons chopped **fresh parsley**

1 tablespoon finely sliced **chives**, or 1 **green onion** (green part only), **thinly sliced**

1 tablespoon **nutritional yeast flakes**

½ teaspoon **dried dill weed**

½ teaspoon **onion powder**

½ teaspoon **garlic granules**

¼ teaspoon **sea salt**

¼ teaspoon freshly ground **black pepper**

BOWLS

4 cups coarsely chopped **leafy greens** (such as stemmed kale, power greens, spinach, or romaine or baby lettuce), **lightly packed**

1 cup shredded **red cabbage**

2 cups cooked **whole grains** (such as barley, brown rice, farro, millet, or quinoa), **cold, warm, or room temperature**

4 slices **Oat Bran–Breaded Tofu** or **Tempeh Cutlets** (page 100), **cut in half lengthwise, then sliced crosswise into thin strips**

1 cup halved **cherry tomatoes** or **grape tomatoes** (preferably a multicolored combination)

1 cup halved and thinly sliced **cucumber** (half-moon slices)

1 cup fresh or frozen **corn,** thawed

¼ cup diced **red onion**

¼ cup toasted **pumpkin seeds,** or 2 tablespoons **hemp seeds**

1   To make the dressing, put all the ingredients in a small bowl and whisk to combine. Let sit for 10 minutes to allow the flavors to blend.

2 Put the leafy greens and cabbage in a small bowl and toss to combine.

3 Use a large, wide bowl or large plate to assemble each of the four servings. For each serving, arrange or layer ½ cup of the whole grains, the strips of 1 tofu cutlet, 1¼ cups of the leafy greens and cabbage mixture, ¼ cup cherry tomatoes, ¼ cup cucumber, ¼ cup corn, 1 tablespoon onion, and 1 tablespoon pumpkin seeds. Drizzle ¼ cup or more of the dressing over the top. Serve immediately.

Save for Later   Stored in separate airtight containers, the ranch dressing, breaded tofu, cooked grains, and other Buddha bowl components will keep for 3 to 5 days in the refrigerator.

BAKED GOODS AND SWEET TREATS

10

FIBER-FILLED oat bran muffins

One of the easiest (and tastiest) ways to work oats and oat bran into your daily diet is by making a batch of these slightly sweet fruit-and-nut muffins, which make a wholesome and filling on-the-go breakfast or snack. The basic muffin recipe is very adaptable; just swap the selection of nuts, dried fruits, and grated fruit or veggies with others that suit your taste and the season.

½ cup plain **oat milk** or other **nondairy milk**

1½ teaspoons **ground flaxseeds** or **flaxseed meal**

¾ cup **oat flour** (see page 45)

½ cup **oat bran**

1½ teaspoons **baking powder**

½ teaspoon **ground cinnamon**

¼ teaspoon **sea salt**

⅓ cup **applesauce**

1½ tablespoons **blackstrap molasses** or **maple syrup**

1 teaspoon **vanilla extract**

¼ cup coarsely grated **apple, carrot,** or **zucchini,** lightly packed

¼ cup **dried fruit** (such as blueberries, cherries, cranberries, chopped dates or prunes, raisins, or a combination)

¼ cup coarsely chopped **raw nuts** or **sunflower seeds**

1 Preheat the oven to 375 degrees F. Line a standard six-cup muffin tin with paper or silicone liners or mist it with cooking spray.

2 Put the milk and flaxseeds in a small bowl and stir to combine. Let sit for 10 minutes to thicken.

3 Put the oat flour, oat bran, baking powder, cinnamon, and salt in a large bowl and stir to combine.

4 Add the flaxseed mixture, applesauce, molasses, and vanilla extract and stir to combine. Gently stir in the apple, dried fruit, and nuts.

5 Fill each muffin cup using ⅓ cup of the batter or until it's three-quarters full or almost level with the top of the liner. Bake for 18 to 20 minutes, until a toothpick inserted in the center of a muffin comes out clean. Let cool in the pan for 5 minutes, then transfer to a rack. Serve warm or room temperature.

Save for Later   Stored in an airtight container, the muffins will keep for 3 days at room temperature or in the refrigerator.

GLUTEN-FREE corn muffins

Makes 6 muffins

A combination of cornmeal, almond flour, and tapioca starch is used in these cornbread muffins, which are lightly sweetened with maple syrup. They are both gluten-free and oil-free, yet they have a moist and tender crumb. Enjoy them with your favorite toppings or spreads or serve them as an accompaniment to chili, soup, or stew or your favorite entrees.

1 cup fine or medium-grind **cornmeal**

1 cup **almond flour**

¼ cup **tapioca starch** or **arrowroot powder**

1 tablespoon **baking powder**

½ teaspoon **sea salt**

1 cup plain **soy milk** or other **nondairy milk**

3 tablespoons plain **oat yogurt** or other **nondairy yogurt**

2 tablespoons **maple syrup** or **agave nectar**

1   Preheat the oven to 375 degrees F. Line a standard six-cup muffin tin with paper or silicone liners or mist it with cooking spray.

2   Put the cornmeal, almond flour, tapioca starch, baking powder, and salt in a large bowl and whisk to combine. Add the milk, yogurt, and maple syrup and whisk to combine.

3   Fill each muffin cup using ⅓ cup of the batter or until it's three-quarters full or almost level with the top of the liner. Bake for 15 to 18 minutes, until a toothpick inserted in the center of a muffin comes out clean. Let cool in the pan for 5 minutes, then transfer to a rack. Serve warm or room temperature.

Variation   **GLUTEN-FREE BLUEBERRY CORN MUFFINS** Gently stir ⅔ cup fresh or frozen blueberries into the finished batter.

Variation

GLUTEN-FREE CORNBREAD Lightly mist an 8-inch round or square baking pan with cooking spray. Spoon the batter into the prepared pan and smooth the top with a silicone spatula. Bake for 20 to 22 minutes, or until the center is set and a toothpick inserted in the center comes out clean.

Save for Later

Stored in an airtight container, the corn muffins or cornbread will keep for 3 days at room temperature or in the refrigerator.

banana, zucchini, and nut BREAD

Makes 1 loaf, 10 slices

Incorporating a wide variety of plant-based foods into your daily meals can help lower LDL cholesterol. This enhanced banana bread makes following that advice easy. It contains potassium-rich bananas, nuts, and chia seeds for omega-3 fatty acids, oat fiber, and zucchini. Who knew that a healthy diet could be so delicious!

2 large **bananas** (preferably overly ripe with brown spots)

½ cup plain **oat milk, almond milk,** or other **nondairy milk**

1 tablespoon **cider vinegar**

1 teaspoon **vanilla extract**

2½ cups **oat flour** (see page 45)

⅓ cup **tapioca starch**

⅓ cup **unbleached cane sugar**

1 tablespoon **chia seeds**

2 teaspoons **baking soda**

½ teaspoon **sea salt**

1¼ cups coarsely grated **zucchini,** lightly packed

⅓ cup coarsely chopped **walnuts** or **hazelnuts**

1 Preheat the oven to 350 degrees F. Line an 8 x 4 x 2½-inch loaf pan with two pieces of parchment paper, overlapping the pieces and allowing the paper to slightly drape over the sides of the pan.

2 Put the bananas, milk, vinegar, and vanilla extract in a food processor and process until light and creamy, 1 minute. Scrape down the work bowl with a silicone spatula and process for 15 seconds longer.

3   Add the oat flour, tapioca starch, sugar, chia seeds, baking soda, and salt and process until smooth, about 1 minute. Scrape down the work bowl with a silicone spatula.

4   Gently squeeze handfuls of the grated zucchini over the sink to remove any excess moisture, then add it to the food processor. Add the walnuts and pulse several times to combine. Spoon the batter into the prepared loaf pan and smooth the top with a silicone spatula.

5   Bake for 45 to 50 minutes, or until a toothpick inserted in the center comes out clean. Let cool in the pan for 20 minutes, then transfer to a rack to cool completely. Serve warm or at room temperature.

Variation   **GARDEN BANANA NUT BREAD**   Decrease the amount of grated zucchini to ⅓ cup and add ⅓ cup coarsely grated carrots, lightly packed (do not squeeze).

Variation   **HEALTHY CHUNKY MONKEY BREAD**   Omit the grated zucchini. Add ¼ cup cacao nibs and ¼ cup unsweetened dried coconut chips or 2 tablespoons unsweetened shredded dried coconut.

Save for Later   Stored in an airtight container, the banana bread will keep for 3 days at room temperature or in the refrigerator.

raspberry fool with aquafaba whipped cream AND ALMOND MERINGUE COOKIES

Makes 4 servings and 12 cookies

This recipe uses Aquafaba Whipped Cream, which does double duty here. Some of the cream is baked to become almond-flavored meringue cookies, and the remainder is swirled with a mixture of wine-infused raspberries and nondairy yogurt to create an refreshing, eye-catching dessert.

ALMOND MERINGUE COOKIES (makes 12 or more cookies)

½ batch (1½ to 2 cups) **Aquafaba Whipped Cream** (page 129)

½ teaspoon **almond extract**

RASPBERRY FOOL

3 cups fresh or frozen **raspberries, thawed**

¼ cup **unbleached cane sugar**

2 tablespoons **red or white wine** (such as Chardonnay, Merlot, Moscato, or Pinot Noir)

1 cup plain **oat yogurt** or other **nondairy yogurt**

½ batch (1½ to 2 cups) **Aquafaba Whipped Cream** (page 129)

¼ cup finely chopped **raw or roasted pistachios**

1. To make the cookies, put the whipped cream and almond extract in a large bowl and whip with electric beaters for 1 minute to evenly distribute the extract.

2. Preheat the oven to 225 degrees F. Line a baking sheet with parchment paper or a silicone baking mat.

3. Portion the meringue mixture onto the lined baking sheet using a 1½-inch ice cream scoop or a heaping tablespoonful for each cookie, spacing them two inches apart.

4 Bake for 60 to 75 minutes, until the tops look and feel dry and are off-white in color. Turn off the oven. Let the cookies cool for 2 hours on the baking sheet in the closed oven.

5 To make the raspberry fool, put the raspberries, sugar, and wine in a medium bowl and stir to combine. Let sit for 15 minutes. Using a fork, coarsely mash the raspberries.

6 Transfer 1 cup of the raspberry mixture to a small bowl. Add the yogurt and stir to combine.

7 To assemble the raspberry fool, put the whipped cream in a medium bowl. Spoon the remaining mashed berries and the raspberry-yogurt mixture in a circular pattern over the top. Using a silicone spatula, fold the mixture twice, turn the bowl one-quarter turn, and fold twice again. Do not overmix; the mixtures should remain as streaks of different colors. Sprinkle the pistachios over the top. Serve the meringue cookies on the side or crushed over the top of individual servings. Serve immediately.

Variation

Replace the raspberries with 3 cups blackberries or sliced strawberries.

Save for Later

Stored in an airtight container or in individual airtight containers, the raspberry fool will keep for 1 day in the refrigerator. Stored in an airtight container, the meringue cookies will keep for several weeks in the refrigerator.

chocolate psyllium pudding PARFAITS

Psyllium husks are the secret ingredient used to thicken the pudding portion of these gorgeous, good-for-you parfaits. Dark cacao powder, bananas, and nut butter are combined with the psyllium husks to create this rich, dark-chocolate treat. The chilled pudding is then sprinkled with a chocolaty crumble made with nuts and dried fruit and topped with fresh fruit, cacao nibs, and dollops of Aquafaba Whipped Cream.

CHOCOLATE CRUMBLE

½ cup **raw or toasted nuts** (such as almonds, hazelnuts, pecans, walnuts, or a combination)

4 pitted **soft dates,** or ¼ cup pitted **soft prunes** or **raisins**

2 tablespoons **unsweetened shredded dried coconut**

2 tablespoons **cacao powder** or **cocoa powder**

PSYLLIUM PUDDING

2 large **bananas** (preferably overly ripe with brown spots)

1⅓ cups plain **almond milk** or other **nondairy milk**

⅓ cup unbleached **cane sugar,** or 3 tablespoons **maple syrup**

2 tablespoons **nut butter** (such as almond, cashew, hazelnut, or peanut)

1 teaspoon **vanilla extract**

1½ tablespoons **psyllium husk powder**

PARFAITS

1 cup whole **raspberries** or sliced **strawberries,** or 1 cup pitted sweet or sour **cherries,** cut in half

¼ cup coarsely chopped **raw or toasted nuts** (such as almonds, hazelnuts, pecans, walnuts, or a combination)

¼ cup **cacao nibs**

1 cup **Aquafaba Whipped Cream** (page 129)

1. To make the chocolate crumble, put all the ingredients in a food processor or blender and process into coarse crumbs. Transfer to a small bowl and set aside.

2. To make the psyllium pudding, put the bananas, milk, sugar, nut butter, and vanilla extract in a food processor or blender and process until smooth. Scrape down the container with a silicone spatula, add the psyllium husk powder, and process for 30 seconds longer. Transfer to a medium bowl and refrigerate until the mixture is very thick and has a pudding-like consistency, 1 hour or longer.

3. Have ready four large glasses or dessert dishes. To assemble each parfait, layer one-quarter of the psyllium pudding in the bottom of each glass or dessert dish. Top the pudding with one-quarter of the chocolate crumble, ¼ cup raspberries, 1 tablespoon chopped nuts, 1 tablespoon cacao nibs, and a large dollop (about ¼ cup) of the whipped cream. Serve immediately.

Save for Later

Stored in an airtight container or individual airtight containers, the psyllium pudding parfaits will keep for 3 days in the refrigerator.

TIP

Using a food processor to make the psyllium pudding results in a creamy, light pudding, and using a blender creates a more airy, mousse-like consistency.

golden milk chia PUDDING

Surprisingly, turmeric, cinnamon, and ginger have antioxidant and anti-inflammatory benefits that have been proven to lower the risk of many illnesses, including heart disease. These colorful spices are combined with coconut milk in the popular Indian beverage known as golden milk, which was the inspiration for this vibrant-yellow chia pudding. It's topped with succulent mango, almonds, coconut, and pomegranate arils.

2 cups plain **coconut milk beverage**

⅓ cup **chia seeds**

2 tablespoons **agave nectar** or **maple syrup**

½ teaspoon **ground ginger**

½ teaspoon **ground turmeric**

¼ teaspoon **ground cinnamon**

¼ teaspoon freshly ground **black pepper**

1 **mango,** peeled and diced

¼ cup **pomegranate arils** or **goji berries**

¼ cup **raw sliced almonds** or **blanched slivered almonds**

¼ cup **unsweetened dried coconut chips,** or 1½ tablespoons **unsweetened shredded dried coconut**

1 Put the coconut milk beverage, chia seeds, agave nectar, ginger, turmeric, cinnamon, and pepper in a small bowl and whisk until well combined. Cover and refrigerate until the chia seeds swell and thicken the mixture into a pudding, 1 hour or longer.

2 Before serving, whisk the mixture to break up any clumps of chia seeds. Top with the mango, pomegranate arils, almonds, and coconut chips. Serve immediately.

Variation | For individual servings, put ½ cup of the pudding in a small bowl, a 10-ounce or larger glass jar, or another small container. Top each serving with one-quarter (about ¼ cup) of the mango and 1 tablespoon each of the pomegranate arils, almonds, and coconut chips.

Save for Later | Stored in an airtight container or individual airtight containers, the chia pudding will keep for 3 days in the refrigerator.

AQUAFABA whipped cream

Makes 3½ to 4 cups

This recipe uses sweetened and whipped aquafaba to create an ultralight creamy topping that resembles whipped cream. Use it to adorn nondairy ice cream sundaes, cakes, or pies. It also makes an amazing egg-free meringue!

¼ cup **aquafaba** (see page 53)

¼ teaspoon **cream of tartar**

½ cup **powdered sugar**

½ teaspoon **vanilla extract**

1. Put a large bowl and electric beaters in the freezer and let chill for 10 minutes.

2. Put the aquafaba and cream of tartar in the chilled bowl. Beat with a mixer on medium speed until soft peaks form, about 5 minutes. Increase to high speed and beat until firm peaks form, about 10 minutes.

3. While still beating, slowly add the powdered sugar and vanilla extract and beat until the cream is glossy and forms very stiff peaks that hold their shape when the beater is lifted, about 5 minutes longer.

Save for Later

Stored in an airtight container, the whipped cream will keep for 3 days in the refrigerator. Over time it may deflate, but it can be whipped again until light and fluffy and stiff peaks form.

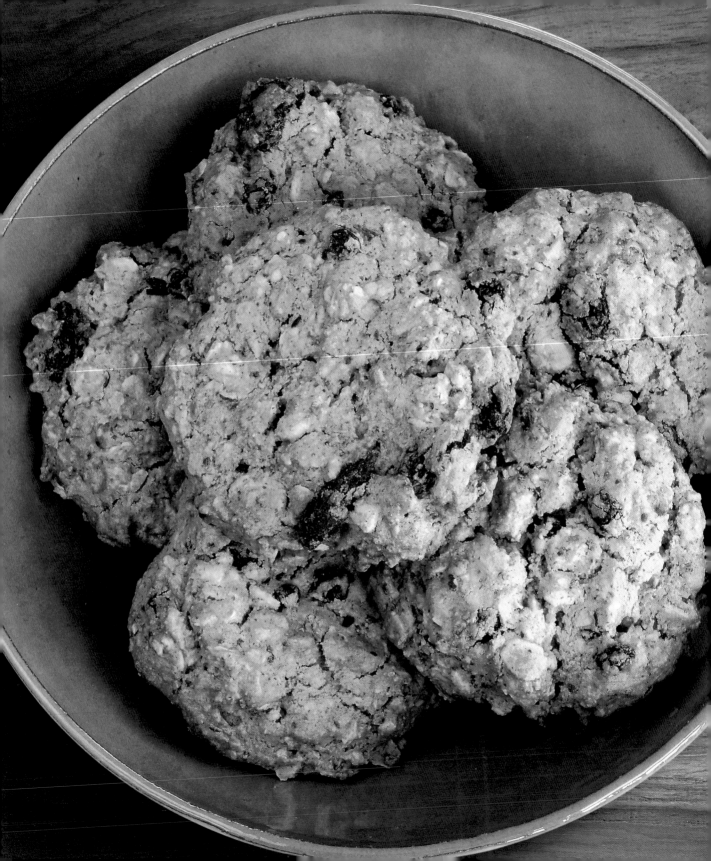

chunky oatmeal and nut butter COOKIES

Rolled oats are a wholesome addition to any cookie dough. These cookies are sweetened with maple syrup and chewy bits of dried fruit, and their richness comes from nut butter, nuts, and seeds. This tasty combination is hard to resist, but try to limit yourself to one or two at a time.

½ cup **maple syrup**

½ cup **nut butter** (such as almond, cashew, peanut, sunflower, or tahini)

¼ cup plain **oat milk** or other **nondairy milk**

1 teaspoon **vanilla extract**

1 cup **oat flour** (see page 45)

2 tablespoons **hemp seeds**

1 tablespoon **chia seeds**

¾ teaspoon **baking powder**

½ teaspoon **baking soda**

½ teaspoon **ground cinnamon**

¼ teaspoon **sea salt**

1⅓ cups **old-fashioned rolled oats**

⅓ cup whole or diced **dried fruit** (such as blueberries, cherries, cranberries, currants, dates, figs, goji berries, mulberries, raisins, or a combination)

⅓ cup coarsely chopped **raw nuts** (such almonds, cashews, hazelnuts, pecans, walnuts, or a combination), **or** ¼ cup raw **sunflower seeds**

1   Preheat the oven to 375 degrees F. Line two baking sheets with parchment paper or a silicone baking mat.

2   Put the maple syrup, nut butter, milk, and vanilla extract in a large bowl and stir to combine. Add the oat flour, hemp seeds, chia seeds, baking powder, baking soda, cinnamon, and salt and stir to combine. Gently stir in the oats, dried fruit, and nuts.

3   Portion the dough onto the lined baking sheets using a 1½-inch ice cream scoop or a heaping tablespoonful for each cookie, spacing them two inches apart. Slightly flatten each cookie with wet fingers.

4   Bake for 10 to 12 minutes, until lightly browned on the bottom and around the edges. Let cool completely on the baking sheets.

Variation   Replace the dried fruit with ¼ cup cacao nibs and ¼ cup unsweetened shredded dried coconut.

Save for Later   Stored in an airtight container, the cookies will keep for 5 days at room temperature or 2 months in the freezer.

gingery peach and berry CRUMBLE

Makes 4 servings

Sliced peaches and plump, juicy berries are lightly spiced and sweetened to make the fruity filling for this old-fashioned dessert, which can be pulled together surprisingly quickly. Serve it plain or topped with a scoop of nondairy ice cream or a dollop of nondairy yogurt or Aquafaba Whipped Cream (page 129) for dessert. Alternatively, top it with a dollop of oat yogurt for a sweet breakfast.

TOPPING

¾ cup old-fashioned **rolled oats**

½ cup coarsely chopped **raw nuts** (such as almonds, hazelnuts, pecans, or walnuts)

¼ cup **raw sunflower seeds**

¼ cup **brown sugar** or **coconut sugar**, lightly packed

¼ cup **maple syrup**

¼ cup **almond flour**

2 tablespoons **unsweetened shredded dried coconut**

½ teaspoon **ground cinnamon**

FRUIT FILLING

3 **peaches**, sliced, or 3 cups sliced frozen peaches (do not thaw)

1½ cups fresh or frozen **blackberries, blueberries,** or **raspberries** (do not thaw)

1 tablespoon peeled and grated **fresh ginger**

2 tablespoons **brown sugar** or **coconut sugar**, lightly packed

2 tablespoons **maple syrup**

2 tablespoons **almond flour**

2 tablespoons **unsweetened shredded dried coconut**

1 teaspoon **ground cinnamon**

1 teaspoon **vanilla extract**

1   Preheat the oven to 375 degrees F. Lightly mist an 8-inch square baking pan with cooking spray.

2   To make the topping, put the oats, nuts, sunflower seeds, brown sugar, maple syrup, almond flour, coconut, and cinnamon in a small bowl and stir to combine.

3 To make the fruit filling, put the peaches, berries, and ginger in a medium bowl. Add the brown sugar, maple syrup, almond flour, coconut, cinnamon, and vanilla extract and stir to combine.

4 Spoon the filling into the prepared baking pan. Sprinkle the oat mixture evenly over the top.

5 Bake for 30 to 35 minutes, until the topping is golden brown and the filling is bubbly. Let cool for 5 minutes before serving. Serve warm or at room temperature.

Variation Replace the sliced peaches with other sliced fruit (such as apples, apricots, nectarines, pears, plums, or pluots).

Save for Later Stored in an airtight container, the crumble will keep for 3 days in the refrigerator.

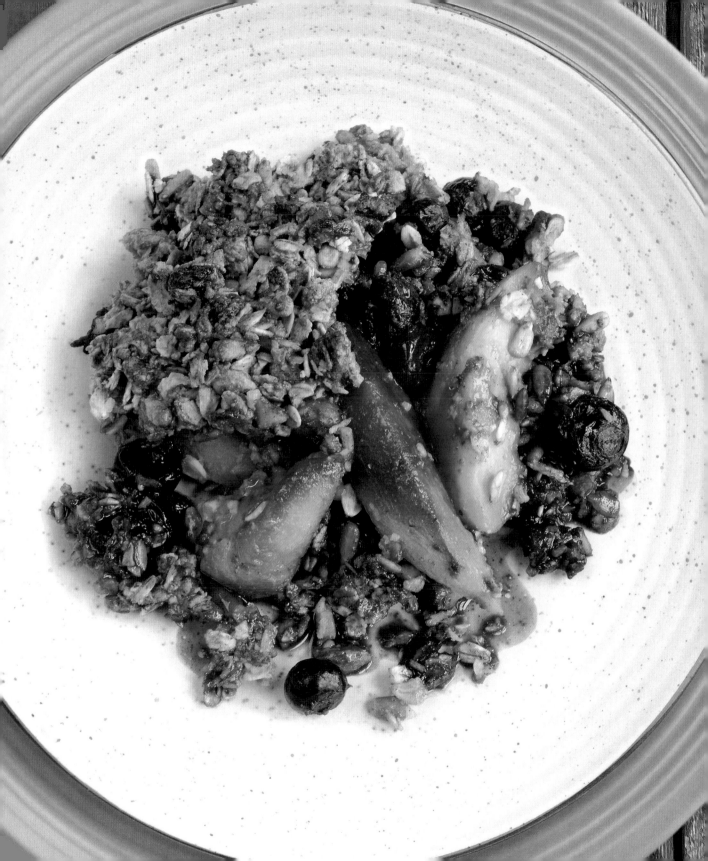

RESOURCES

Astro-CHARM

astrocharm.org/calculator

This app assists patients and health-care providers in estimating the ten-year risk of atherosclerotic cardiovascular disease (ASCVD), incorporating traditional cardiovascular risk factors as well as coronary artery calcium (CAC) score values.

FH Foundation

thefhfoundation.org

This patient-centered nonprofit organization is dedicated to the research, advocacy, and education of familial hypercholesterolemia (FH) in order to increase the rate of early diagnosis and encourage proactive treatment. For the FH Foundation's list of lipoprotein apheresis centers in the US and Canada, visit https://thefhfoundation.org/diagnosis-management/treatment-for-hofh/lipoprotein-apheresis-centers.

Lipoprotein(a) Foundation

lipoproteinafoundation.org

This national nonprofit organization provides general information about lipoprotein(a).

SHAPE (Society for Heart Attack Prevention and Eradication)

shapesociety.org

This nonprofit organization promotes public and professional education for early detection of individuals with atherosclerotic plaques who are at risk of heart attack and stroke but have no symptoms.

REFERENCES

Chapter 1

Berg K. A new serum type system in man—the Lp system. *Acta Pathol Microbiol Scand.* 1963;59:369–82.

Enas EA et al. Lipoprotein(a): An independent, genetic, and causal factor for cardiovascular disease and acute myocardial infarction. *Indian Heart J.* 2019 Mar-Apr;71(2):99–112.

Ergou S et al. Lipoprotein(a) concentration and the risk of coronary heart disease, stroke, and nonvascular mortality. *JAMA.* 2009 Jul 22;302(4):412–23.

Wang Z et al. Prognostic value of lipoprotein (a) level in patients with coronary artery disease: a meta-analysis. *Lipids Health Dis.* 2019 Jul 8;18(1):1092–6.

Kampstrup PR et al. Genetically elevated lipoprotein(a) and increased risk of myocardial infarction. *JAMA.* 2009 Jun 10;301(22):2331–9.

Hippe DS et al. Lp(a) (lipoprotein(a)) levels predict progression of carotid atherosclerosis in subjects with atherosclerotic cardiovascular disease on intensive lipid therapy. *Arterioscler Thromb Vasc Biol.* 2018 Mar;38(3):673–678.

Nave AH et al. Lipoprotein (a) as a risk factor for ischemic stroke: a meta-analysis. *Atherosclerosis.* 2015 Oct;242(2):496–503.

Beheshtian A et al. Lipoprotein (a) level, apolipoprotein (a) size, and risk of unexplained ischemic stroke in young and middle-aged adults. *Atherosclerosis.* 2016 Oct;253:47–53.

Kamstrup PR et al. Elevated lipoprotein(a) and risk of aortic valve stenosis in the general population. *J Am Coll Cardiol.* 2014 Feb 11;63(5):470–7.

Thanassoulis G et al. Genetic associations with valvular calcification and aortic stenosis. *N Engl J Med.* 2013 Feb 7;368(6):503–12.

Costello BT et al. Lipoprotein(a) and increased cardiovascular risk in women. *Clin Cardiol.* 2016 Feb;39(2):96–102.

Orth-Gomer K et al. Lipoprotein(a) as a determinant of coronary heart disease in young women. *Circulation.* 1997 Jan 21;95(2):329–34.

McNeal CJ. Lipoprotein(a): Its relevance to the pediatric population. *J Clin Lipidol.* 2015 Sep–Oct;9(5 Suppl):S57–66.

Vanuzzo D. The epidemiological concept of residual risk. *Intern Emerg Med.* 2011 Oct;6 Suppl 1:45–51.

Cai A et al. Lipoprotein(a): a promising marker for residual cardiovascular risk assessment. *Dis Markers.* 2013;35(5):551–9.

Zhao Y. Session 4: Young Investigator Presentations. Model predicts 5-year ASCVD risk in patients on statin therapy. American Society for Preventive Cardiology Congress on CVD Prevention, San Antonio, TX. July 19–21, 2019.

Tsamikas S et al. NHLBI working group recommendations to reduce lipoprotein(a)-mediated risk of cardiovascular disease and aortic stenosis. *J Am Coll Cardiol.* 2018 Jan 16;71(2):177–192.

Han L et al. National trends in American Heart Association revised Life's Simple 7 metrics associated with risk of mortality among US adults. *JAMA Netw Open.* 2019 Oct 2;2(10):e1913131.

Ford ES et al. Ideal cardiovascular health and mortality from all causes and diseases of the circulatory system among adults in the United States. *Circulation.* 2012;125(8):987–995.

Mozzafarian D et al. Heart disease and stroke statistics—2016 update. A report from the American Heart Association. *Circulation.* 2016;133:e38–360.

Wilson DP et al. Use of lipoprotein(a) in clinical practice: A biomarker whose time has come. A scientific statement from the National Lipid Association. *J Clin Lipidol.* 2019 May–Jun;13(3):374–92.

Task Force Members. 2019 ESC/EAS guidelines for the management of dyslipidaemias: Lipid modification to reduce cardiovascular risk. *Atherosclerosis.* 2019;S0021.

Blood tests to determine risk of coronary artery disease. The Cleveland Clinic. Last revised September, 30, 2019. my.clevelandclinic.org/health/diagnostics/16792-blood-tests-to-determine-risk-of-coronary-artery-diseases.

Benjamin EJ et al. Heart disease and stroke statistics—2019 update: a report from the American Heart Association. *Circulation.* January 31, 2019.

Heart Disease Fact Sheet. Centers for Disease Control and Prevention. https://www.cdc.gov/dhdsp/data_statistics/fact_sheets/fs_heart_disease.htm.

Chapter 2

Tsimikas S. A test in context: lipoprotein(a): diagnosis, prognosis, controversies, and emerging therapies. *J Am Coll Cardiol.* 2017 Feb 14;69(6):692–711.

Yeang C et al. Effect of therapeutic interventions on oxidized phospholipids on apolipoprotein B100 and lipoprotein(a). *J Clin Lipidol*. 2016 May–Jun;10(3):594–603.

Tsimikas S et al. Statin therapy increases lipoprotein(a) levels. *Eur Heart J*. 2019 May 20;pii:ehz310.

van Wissen S et al. Long term statin treatment reduces lipoprotein(a) concentrations in heterozygous familial hypercholesterolaemia. *Heart*. 2003 Aug;89(8):893–6.

Wilson DP et al. Use of lipoprotein(a) in clinical practice: A biomarker whose time has come. A scientific statement from the National Lipid Association. *J Clin Lipidol*. 2019 May–Jun;13(3):374–92.

Cook NR et al. Lipoprotein(a) and cardiovascular risk prediction among women. *J Am Coll Cardiol*. 2018 Jul 17;72(3):287–296.

Sahebkar A et al. Comparison of the effects of fibrates versus statins on plasma lipoprotein(a) concentrations: a systematic review and meta-analysis of head-to-head randomized controlled trials. *BMC Med*. 2017 Feb. 3;15(1):22.

Sahebkar A et al. Impact of ezetimibe on plasma lipoprotein(a) concentrations as monotherapy or in combination with statins: a systematic review and meta-analysis of randomized controlled trials. *Sci Rep*. 2018 Dec 14;8(1):17887.

Helmbold AF et al. The effects of extended release niacin in combination with omega 3 fatty acid supplements in the treatment of elevated lipoprotein (a). *Cholesterol*. 2010;306:147.

Santos HO et al. Lipoprotein(a): current evidence for a physiologic role and the effects of nutraceutical strategies. *Clin Ther*. 2019 Sep;41(9):1780–1797.

Penson P et al. Does coffee consumption alter plasma lipoprotein(a) concentrations? A systematic review. *Crit Rev Food Sci Nutr*. 2018 July 3;58(10):1706–1714.

Singh RB, Niaz MA. Serum concentration of lipoprotein(a) decreases on treatment with hydrosoluble coenzyme Q10 in patients with coronary artery disease: discovery of a new role. *Int J Cardiol*. 1999 Jan;68(1):23–9.

Shojaei M et al. Effects of carnitine and coenzyme Q10 on lipid profile and serum levels of lipoprotein(a) in maintenance hemodialysis patients on statin therapy. *Iran J Kidney Dis*. 2011 Mar;5(2):114–8.

Sahebkar A et al. Supplementation with coenzyme Q10 reduces plasma lipoprotein(a) concentrations but not other lipid indices: A systematic review and meta-analysis. *Pharmacol Res*. 2016 Mar;105:198–209.

Sirtori CR et al. L-carnitine reduces plasma lipoprotein(a) levels in patients with hyper Lp(a). *Nutr Metab Cardiovasc Dis*. 2000 Oct;10(5):247–51.

Serban MC et al. Impact of L-carnitine on plasma lipoprotein(a) concentrations: A systematic review and meta-analysis of randomized controlled trials. *Sci Rep*. 2016 Jan 12;6:19188.

Vallance HD et al. Marked elevation in plasma trimethylamine-N-oxide (TMAO) in patients with mitochondrial disorders treated with oral L-carnitine. *MGM Reports.* 2008;15:130–133.

Rath M, Pauling L. Hypothesis: lipoprotein(a) is a surrogate for ascorbate. *Proc Natl Acad Sci USA.* 1990 Aug;87(16):6204–7.

Cha J et al. Hypoascorbemia induces atherosclerosis and vascular deposition of lipoprotein(a) in transgenic mice. *Am J Cardiovasc Dis.* 2015 Mar 20;5(1):53–62.

Anagnostis P et al. The effect of hormone replacement therapy and tibolone on lipoprotein (a) concentrations in postmenopausal women. *Maturitas.* 2017 May;99:27–36.

Soma MR et al. The lowering of lipoprotein[a] induced by estrogen plus progesterone replacement therapy in postmenopausal women. *Arch Int Med.* 1993 Jun 28; 153(12):1462–8.

Suk Danik J et al. Lipoprotein(a), hormone replacement therapy, and risk of future cardiovascular events. *J Am Coll Cardiol.* 2008 Jul 8;52(2):124–31.

Zmunda JM et al. Testosterone decreases lipoprotein(a) in men. *Am J Cardiol.* 1996 Jun 1;77(14):1244–7.

O'Donoghue ML et al. Lipoprotein(a), PCSK9 inhibition, and cardiovascular risk. *Circulation.* 2019 Mar 19;139(12):1483–1492.

Schettler VJJ et al. Lipoprotein apheresis is an optimal therapeutic option to reduce increased Lp(a) levels. *Clin Res Cardiol Suppl.* 2019 Apr;14(Suppl 1):33–38.

Heigl F et al. Efficacy, safety, and tolerability of long-term lipoprotein apheresis in patients with LDL- or Lp(a) hyperlipoproteinemia. *Atheroscler Suppl.* 2015 May;18:154–62.

Khan TZ et al. Apheresis as novel treatment for refractory angina with raised lipoprotein(a): a randomized controlled cross-over trial. *Eur Heart J.* 2017 May 21;38(20): 1561–1569.

Khan TZ et al. Impact of lipoprotein apheresis on thrombotic parameters in patients with refractory angina and raised lipoprotein(a). *J Clin Lipidol.* 2019 Sep-Oct;13(5):788–796.

Tsimikas S et al. LBS.02—Novel approaches to CV prevention. American Heart Association Scientific Sessions, Chicago IL. Nov. 10–12, 2018.

Chapter 3

Clevidence BA et al. Plasma lipoprotein (a) levels in men and women consuming diets enriched in saturated, cis-, or trans-monounsaturated fatty acids. *Arterioscler Thromb Vasc Biol.* 1997 Sep;17(9):1657–61.

Haring B et al. Healthy dietary interventions and lipoprotein (a) plasma levels: results from the Omni Heart Trial. *PLoS One.* 2014 Dec 15;9(12):e114859.

Najjar R et al. Consumption of a defined, plant-based diet reduces lipoprotein(a), inflammation, and other atherogenic lipoproteins and particles within 4 weeks. *Clin Cardiol*. 2018 Aug;41(8):1062–8.

Bloedon LT et al. Flaxseed and cardiovascular risk factors: results from a double blind, randomized, controlled clinical trial. *J Am Coll Nutr*. 2008 Feb;27(1):65–74.

Anderson JW et al. Oat-bran cereal lowers serum total and LDL cholesterol in hyper-cholesterolemic men. *Am J Clin Nutrition*. 1990 Sep;52:495–99.

Kristensen M, Bugel S. A diet rich in oat bran improves blood lipids and hemostatic factors, and reduces apparent energy digestibility in young healthy volunteers. *Eur J Clin Nutrit*. 2011 Jun;65:1053–1058.

Perrot N et al. Ideal cardiovascular health influences cardiovascular disease risk associated with high lipoprotein(a) levels and genotype: The EPIC-Norfolk prospective population study. *Atherosclerosis*. 2017 Jan;256:47–52.

Mackinnon LT et al. Effects of physical activity and diet on lipoprotein(a). *Med Sci Sports Exerc*. 1997 Nov;29(11):1429-36.

Morrison LM. Reductions of mortality rate in coronary atherosclerosis by a low cholesterol-low fat diet. *Am Heart J*. 1951 Oct;42(4):538–45.

Pritikin N. The Pritikin Diet. *JAMA*. 1984;251(9):1160–1.

Ornish D et al. Intensive lifestyle changes for reversal of coronary heart disease. *JAMA*. 1998 Dec 16;280(23):1–7.

Esselstyn CB Jr et al. A way to reverse CAD? *J Fam Practice*. 2014 Jul;63(7):356–64.

Martinez-Gonzales MA et al. A provegetarian food pattern and reductions in total mortality in the PREDIMED study. *Am J Clin Nutr*. 2014 Jul;100 Suppl 1:320S–8S.

Kim H et al. Plant-based diets are associated with a lower risk of incident cardiovascular disease, cardiovascular disease mortality, and all-cause mortality in a general population of middle-aged adults. *J Am Heart Assoc*. 2019 Aug;8:1–13.

Alshahrani SM et al. Red and processed meat and mortality in a low meat intake population. *Nutrients*. 2019 Mar 14;11(3):E622.

Guasch-Ferre M et al. Meta-analysis of randomized controlled trials of red meat consumption in comparison with various comparison diets on cardiovascular risk factors. *Circulation*. 2019 Aug 9;139(15):1828–1845.

Jenkins DJ et al. The effect of a plant-based low-carbohydrate ("Eco-Atkins") diet on body weight and blood lipid concentrations in hyperlipidemic subjects. *Arch Intern Med*. 2009 Jun 8;169(11):1046–54.

GBD 2017 Diet Collaborators. Health effects of dietary risks in 195 countries, 1990–2017. *Lancet*. 2019 Apr;393:1958–1972.

Virtanen HEK et al. Dietary proteins and protein sources and risk of death: the Kuopio Ischaemic Heart Disease Risk Factor Study. *Am J Clin Nutr.* 2019 May 1;109(5):1462–1471.

Bradbury KE et al. Diet and colorectal cancer in UK Biobank: a prospective study. *Int J Epidemiol.* 2019 Apr 17;64:1–13.

Genoni A et al. Long-term paleolithic diet is associated with lower resistant starch intake, different gut microbiota composition and increased serum TMAO concentrations. *Eur J Nutr.* 2019 Jul 5;17:1–14.

Kawanishi K, et al. Human species-specific loss of CMP-N-acetylneuraminic acid hydroxylase enhances atherosclerosis via intrinsic and extrinsic mechanism. *PNAS.* 2019 Aug 6; 116(32):16036–16045.

Wilson JM et al. IgE to the mammalian oligosaccharide galactose-α-1,3-galactose is associated with increased atheroma volume and plaques with unstable characteristics-brief report. *Arterioscl Thromb Vasc Biol.* 2018 Jul;38(7):1665–1669.

ABOUT THE AUTHORS

JOEL K. KAHN, MD, is a clinical professor of medicine at Wayne State University School of Medicine. Known as America's Healthy Heart Doc, he is a contributor to many online sites, such as LinkedIn and Thrive Global, and has appeared several times on the *Dr. Phil* and *The Doctors* television shows. Dr. Kahn founded the Kahn Center for Cardiac Longevity and owns GreenSpace & Go in Royal Oak, Michigan. He is also the author of *The Plant-Based Solution, Dead Execs Don't Get Bonuses*, and *Vegan Sex.* Visit drjoelkahn.com.

BEVERLY LYNN BENNETT is a seasoned vegan chef and baker, writer, and animal advocate, who is passionate about showing the world how easy, delicious, and healthy it is to follow a plant-based diet. Beverly can often be found at Northwest regional VegFests doing food demos. She is the author of more than a dozen cookbooks, including *The Anti-Inflammatory Cookbook, Spiralize!*, and *The Complete Idiot's Guide to Vegan Cooking.*

Acknowledgments

From Joel K. Kahn, MD

I want to thank the amazing team and patients at the Kahn Center for Cardiac Longevity for their trust in advanced heart care and the ability to work toward preventing and reversing cardiovascular disease.

From Beverly Lynn Bennett

My deepest gratitude to Joel Kahn, MD, for asking me to be a part of this book and for shining a spotlight on lipoprotein(a). On a personal level, I was eager to learn more about the inherited risk, as several of my family members have battled heart disease. Working on this book with Dr. Kahn also provided me with a way of honoring my dad, who recently lost his battle with pancreatic cancer and heart disease, and I know that he would be eager to read this book and proud of me for being a part of it.

My sincerest thanks to everyone at Book Publishing Company, especially to Bob Holzapfel for having the insight to pair me with Dr. Kahn for this project. I am also grateful to Managing Editor Jo Stepaniak for once again working her editorial magic, to Alan Roettinger for the food styling and photos, and to Michael Thomas for pulling everything together.

Finally, I'm eternally thankful to my husband, Ray Sammartano, for all of his love and understanding, and for encouraging me when I need it most. We went vegetarian independently in our teens and started our vegan journey together in our twenties. I deeply appreciate his support of my work as a vegan cookbook author and his honesty as my loyal sounding board, grammar guru, and recipe taste-tester for all of the books that I've written.

INDEX

greens, beer-braised, with black-eyed peas, as variation, 79
Green Smoothie, Cherry Cobbler, 35
Green Tea, Melon, and Mango Smoothie, 33
Guacamole, Black Bean, Sweet Potatoes Loaded with, 82–83

H

Harper, Bob, 1
Harvard School of Public Health studies, 25
healthy chunky monkey bread, as variation, 123
heart (cardiovascular) disease
  age and, 7, 9, 11, 16, 29
  apheresis to treat, 19
  detecting, 9–12
  diet and, 11, 20, 22, 23
  Esselstyn, Caldwell, and, 24
  Finnish study and, 26
  genes/genetics and, 9, 11
  Harper, Bob, and, 1
  heart murmur and, 9, 29
  hormone replacement therapy (HRT) and, 18
  Life's Simple 7 and, 5
  lifestyle and, 27
  Lp(a) and, 1, 2, 3, 5, 7, 20, 22
  Morrison, Lester, and, 23
  Neu5Gc and, 27
  omega-3 fatty acids and, 18
  Ornish, Dean, and, 24
  plant-based diet and, 25, 28
  primer about, 10–11
  Pritikin, Nathan, and, 24
  red meat consumption and, 16–17, 25, 26, 27
  as reversible, 20, 21
  risks/risk assessment and, 4–5, 10–11, 18, 21, 22, 25, 26
  as silent disease, v
  statins and, 14

stroke(s) and, 9, 10
studies about, 3, 4
tick bites and, 27
vitamin C and, 17
HeFH (heterozygous familial hyperlipidemia), 14
hemp
  and Almond Parmesan, 50
  Falafel Burgers, 96–97
  Hemp Seed, Avocado, and Spinach Pesto, 51
heterozygous familial hyperlipidemia (HeFH), 14
high blood pressure, 2, 3, 11, 24
high Lp(a), 3–4, 29–32
hormone replacement therapy (HRT), 18
HRT (hormone replacement therapy), 18
Hummus, Beet, 55

I

INTERHEART study, 3

J

Jenkins, David, 25
Journal of the American Heart Association, 25

K

Kale (Tuscan) and Brussels Sprouts Caesar Salad with Lemon-Tahini Dressing, 75–76
Kidney Bean, Corn, and Quinoa Chili, 59–60

L

The Lancet, 24
L-carnitine to reduce Lp(a), 15, 16–17, 31
LDL cholesterol
  apheresis and, 18–19
  diet and, 14

ezetimibe and, 15
lifestyle and, 31–32
PCSK9 inhibitors and, 18–19
plant-based diets and, 21–22, 25–26
residual risk and, 5
size and, 2
statins and, 14, 31
tests/testing and, 7, 8, 30
therapies and, 29, 31–32
Lemony Pasta with Artichokes, Beans, and Spinach, 110–111
lentil(s)
  and Rice Pilaf, 90–91
  and rice pilaf, celebration, as variation, 91
  in soup recipes, 64–65, 66–67
Life's Simple 7, 6, 22
lifestyle and Lp(a), 2, 5, 11, 20–22
Lime and Chile Dressing, Red, Black and Blue Fruit Salad with, 37
lysine, 16, 17, 30–31

M

main dishes
  Bean and Rice Burritos, 98–99
  Chestnut, Roasted, and Mushroom Bourguignon, 104–105
  Grain and Garden Buddha Bowls with Yogurt Ranch Dressing, 115–116
  Hemp Falafel Burgers, 96–97
  Millet, Cheesy, and Vegetable Casserole with Almond Crumb Topping, 112–113
  Pasta, Lemony, with Artichokes, Beans, and Spinach, 110–111
  Ratatouille, 106
  Sheet-Pan Supper, 102–103
  Tempeh Bolognese with Mushrooms and Red Wine, 108–109
  Tofu or Tempeh Cutlets, Oat Bran-Breaded, 100–101

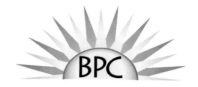

books that educate, inspire, and empower

To find your favorite books on plant-based cooking and nutrition,
raw-foods cuisine, and healthy living, visit:

BookPubCo.com

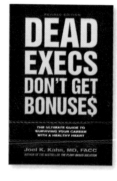
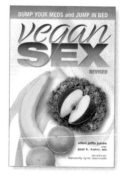
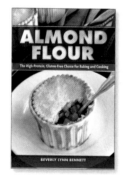
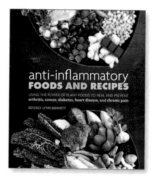